BOOK OF SPIRIT
VOLUME TWO

ADULT PRAYER

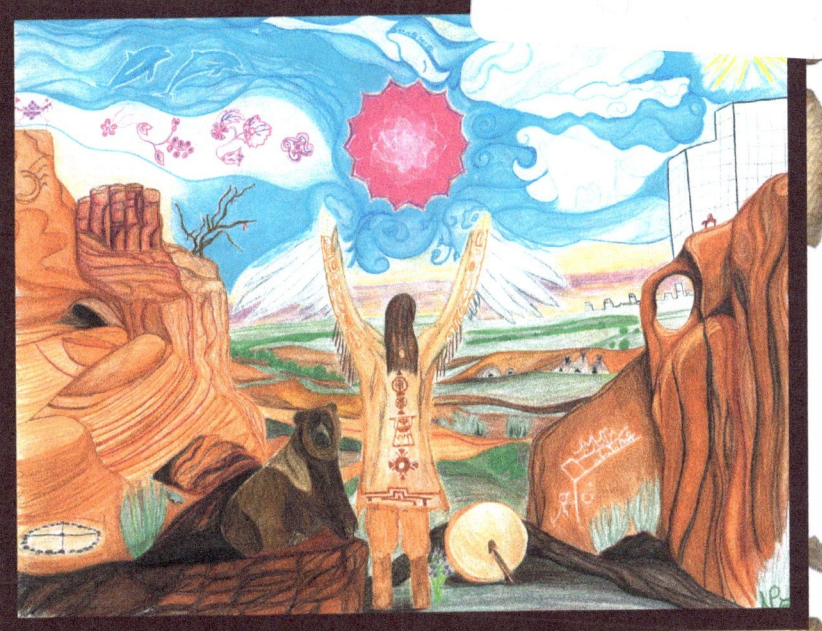

From a Healer's Eye

Written By William Two Feather

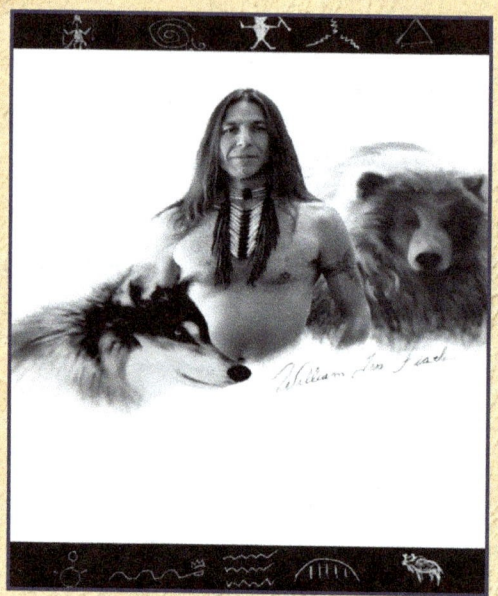

Two Feather

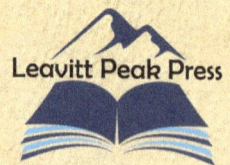

Leavitt Peak Press

ISBN: 978-1-967361-76-2 (sc)
ISBN: 978-1-967361-60-1 (e)

The underlying thread we weave with is,
as Grandmother Spider Woman would say,
"In a good way and with a good heart"

PERSONAL MEDICINE STATEMENT

I, William Two Feather, sit here today, pen in hand, fully aware of the gravity of knowledge that has been passed down from many generations of experience. This line of service "for the people," was not my choice ~ it was chosen for me. My teachers were not sought out, however they came in time.

There are several reasons for wearing the moccasins of healer/ teacher today. Many years ago, three teachers of high standing in the Turtle Island (indigenous) people's medicine world, personally tested me for a year each. Then came the day of formal acceptance as an apprentice and so the long journey began (so it seemed back then.)

After about ten years of apprenticeship, it was time to get on with it, so the first leg of the journey began within the United States. This time of being in service brought clarity into existence for the healer, lecturer, and teacher. After six or seven years, the day came to travel across the pond to Europe, and then to the lands below the Equator. Professional faith healing brought me to many countries, and with the use of translators, many students have given me the great honor and blessing of calling me, 'Teacher.'

All of this has provided me the life experience and wisdom to put to pen and paper these experiences and teachings for you.

Long ago (several decades) those who have taught me what I know said this, "You have been chosen to write down oral tradition. Do not read any books on these topics. We will instruct you." Their expressed concern was that in these fast times there was the danger of this Spiritual knowledge going six feet under the ground with them.

This book is part of a series of 7 books containing Native American teachings as well as the teachings of other indigenous peoples of the Earth. Each of these books are designed to be a journey unto themselves.

AHO ~ William Two Feather
Pray with a good heart and in a good way!
Walk in beauty.

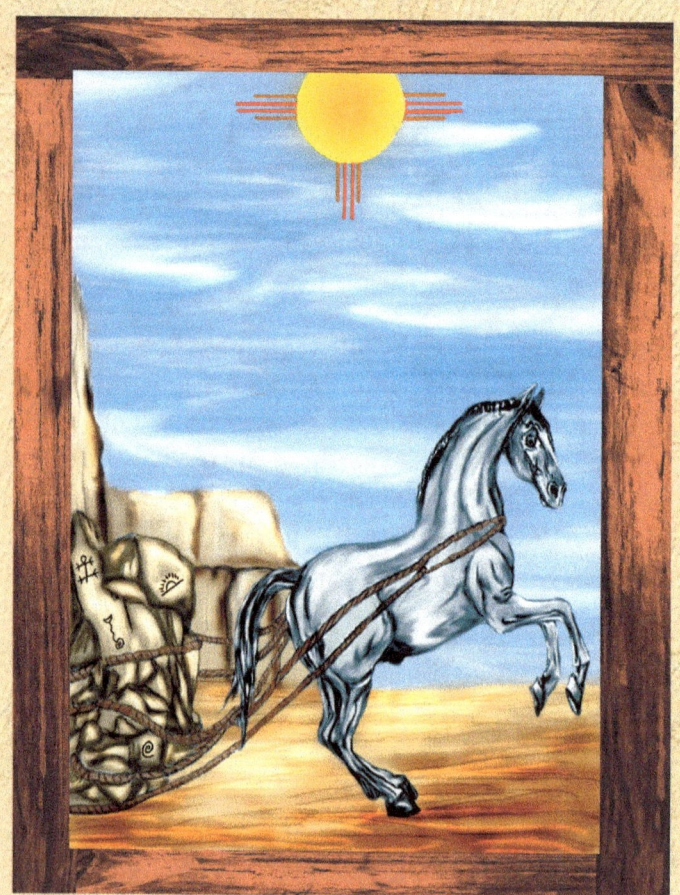

Strength

CONTENTS

PRAYER

Prayer has been with us from ancient times, before the written word, even before formal languages were around.

Prayer has had mystical connotations and magical qualities attributed to it since time began.

Prayer has turned out to be one of the strongest allies in continuing to spread light throughout the world, to keep the balance, and to foster harmony and tolerance.

Prayer is something that exceeds all language and cultural barriers, and is an accepted practice in all cultures.

The Power of Prayer

The power of prayer is very strong, and goes farther than most know. It has the power to lift the spirits, strengthen the weak, heal the sick and revive self-esteem. Prayer serves us in all our needs.

The ancient type of prayer is done mostly with gestures that symbolically mimic the environment as well as the realm of Spirit.

The Power of The Word

There are three different methods of prayer empowerment:
* The Spoken Word
* The Written Word
* The Unspoken Word

Using "The Power of the Word" method is one of the best ways to maximize the petitioner's endeavours to have their prayers tended to.

The more the seeker becomes familiar with other aspects of prayer, with Indigenous peoples' beliefs and with their histories of prayer, the more knowledge the seeker has to draw upon to use prayer in a good way and with a good heart.

It gives us more tools at our beck and call, if we choose to use them.

This book draws on Native American ways as its' basic foundation; however, the belief systems of many other Indigenous cultures are intricately woven throughout the fabric of these teachings, if it works.

The ultimate goal is to bring forth Indigenous teachings because this is the time before change in the world. It has been said in Native American prophecies that certain signs would be shown and then would come Earth changes. These prayer teachings are meant to be shared with those who seek to know them, yet who may not have access in any other way.

As a healer who travels the world in a professional capacity living this way, I can assure you that there is more to this than meets the eye. There is a key here for those who choose to use it. This book is written on more than one level:

+ The words on the page
+ What is written between the lines
+ What only 2% of readers will get (and if you have to ask what that is then it is not yet your time to understand)

As spiritual beings, we have certain truths to assist us in our attempt to be in harmony with ourselves and to be conscious of our environment. We cannot simply pick and choose what we should or should not abide by when it comes to spirit. You have the power and authority to decide on a course of action for your life and then you should stick with it.

When a lifestyle has been committed to, then that is what it is. When in doubt ask your heart.

It is common practice, and convenient, to ask someone else for the answers to the difficult questions of life. However, you could use the "looks with-in" medicine of the bear[1] and find your own answers, since all things reside within you.

Spirit works in many ways. As a youth I can remember my dad saying, "Hold out your hand and ask for what you want." He was telling me that I needed to make the effort if I wanted things to get done.

One day while making a personal medicine wheel way up in the mountains, I asked Spirit this question; "How do I initiate communications with the world of spirit?"

The answer that came back to me was metaphorical: "If you were to throw a ball at a target to hit a bulls-eye, I, spirit, cannot hit the target for you until you pick up the ball and throw it."[2]

In this is a deep teaching, but just in case it was too deep, here is a tip: both dark and light can do such things. So in a spiritual situation, it is advisable to be the initiator; spirit has a very difficult time doing anything about your request if you don't make the request discernible. Simply put it out there to the universe. "I accept this assistance as long as it comes in a good way and with a good heart, and hurts no one or no thing."

---

[1] *Bear medicine is also called "looks with-in" medicine. What does a bear do in the winter? Hibernates, and in so doing is with himself for a long period of time, allowing much looking-within time. When you use this medicine, ask for something specific.*
[2] *To know this is to grasp the first of the three levels this book of spirit has to share: that we are not only ourselves, but are a part of all our relatives, and that what we do has an influence on all our relatives.*

A STORY OF INDIVIDUAL MEDICINE

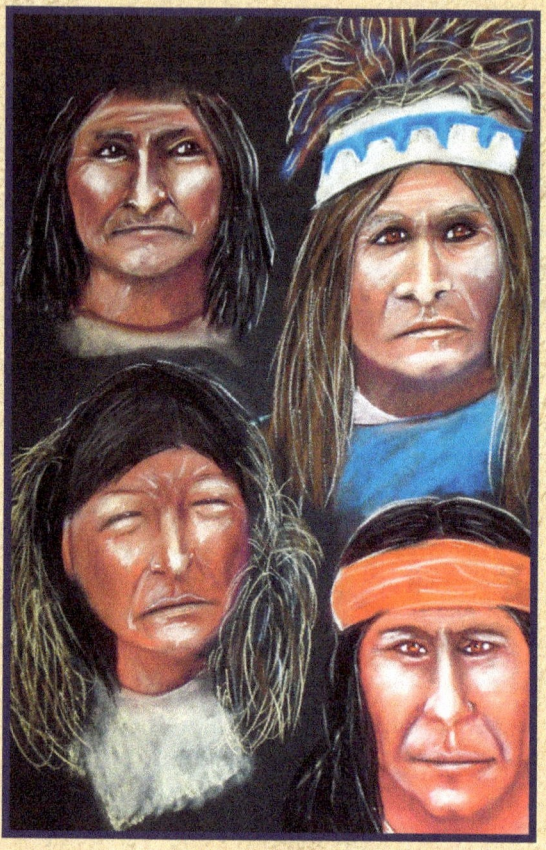

Elders

This reminds me of a nice traditional story. Know that these stories have been told for many generations and now come to those who ask to know them.

There was an old woman and an old man: Grandmother was white haired and so was Grandfather. They had raised their young ones and had taken places of respect in their community. However, Grandmother soon grew restless. She missed the times of having to feed a whole bunch at every meal, and all the other nice things she had done to tend to the needs of a nest full of children. So she got an idea to go out into the forest and look for some medicine. She had never received any formal healing training and now wanted to become a healer, and be of assistance.

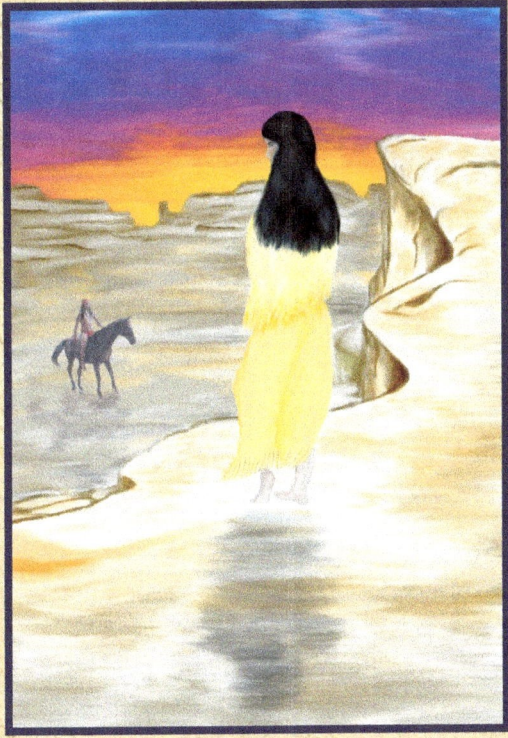

Lovers

She discussed the situation with her other half[3] and they decided it was something that would be done. Her idea was to go out into the woods for four days, very far away from the place where they had lived for so long a time. She would walk for a few days, then find a special place and begin her fast and prayers.

She walked and walked, and this was a short round

---

[3] *Other Half is a common reference to an Indian marriage. The husband and wife lead separate lives until marriage when they walk the same trail as one.*

Grandmother with long white hair[4], but she was strong. Finally, she found the spot, and it was not beautiful at all, but Grandmother felt very comfortable there. She had blazed many trails in her long walk on the medicine wheel of life and had picked up a thing or two along the way.

Grandmother began to purify herself to prepare for the next four days of fasting (no food or water) and many prayers. The quest was to go and get Bear Medicine so she could use it to start doing healing work.

She prayed for three days, yet no bear came to give her the blessing of teaching her how this medicine worked and how to use it to serve others in a good way and with a good heart.

By the fourth day, Grandmother was beside herself. Realizing that she was not to receive Bear Medicine, she slowly got up from her difficult fast. When she got to her knees, she really felt her advanced age.

The way back home was difficult, but she plugged on until her home was in sight. It was a bittersweet moment. When Grandmother reached her door, she was shocked! Sitting in her place eating her dinner with her other half was Mr. Bear.

No words were said. Mr. Bear simply stood up, dismissed himself with a nod of the head to Grandfather and left, without acknowledging Grandmother in the slightest. Oh, Grandmother was really not happy now, and slowly went to her bed and had a bowl of soup her husband prepared and brought for her.

It was not long before things at home deteriorated to a not very happy place. So Grandmother figured she would give it another attempt. Her rationale was that since she had chosen

---

[4] It is believed by many tribes that the hair contains our spirit, and the longer the hair, the closer the connection to our Mother, the Earth. It is a big offense to touch any Indian's hair without asking permission.

the medicine animal herself, she must have chosen the wrong animal, had not stayed long enough, nor prayed hard enough. The next trip would be even farther away and she would pray harder and fast for eight days this time.

So off she went, walking for many more days to seek out Eagle Medicine[5], perceiving this to be the medicine she was meant to receive.

When she finally reached her destination, the land was very strange to her. She set up her own individual medicine wheel[6] and began to pray. For the first few days, she did a little dance to greet Grandfather Sun when he rose in the morning and set at night. The fast was really taking a toll on this old Grandmother, but she was adamant about receiving her medicine so she stuck to the plan.

It was so difficult; nevertheless, she knew it was our way to sacrifice much in seeking medicine. She kept fasting and praying, long and hard, yet nothing she did seemed to bring any Eagle Medicine.

By the end of eight days, she could hardly get to her knees. Realizing that Mrs. Eagle was not going to come and give her a blessing about how to use such medicine, Grandmother got bitter and started to crawl until she was able to get to her feet and walk toward home at a very slow and painful pace.

As Grandmother got closer to her house, the hardship she had endured was so unbearable she collapsed. In agony, she picked

---

[5] Eagle Medicine is that of the messenger, of truth and of new beginnings. This is the medicine of the East, the direction where the Grandmothers and Grandfathers share this powerful medicine.

[6] Individual Medicine Wheel: There are many types of medicine wheels that are used for different times and purposes. One is for time keeping, personal healing, personal questions, spiritual journeying, discovery etc. This particular medicine wheel is for seeking of spiritual council. This is our traditional honoring and teaching chalkboard school house all rolled up in one place in four directions.

her wretched self up from the ground and dragged herself to the door. When she saw who was in her house having her dinner with her half-side, she was aghast.

Yes, Grandmother. Mr. Eagle hopped to attention, gave his respects to his host with a nod of his head and went for the door. He politely gave Grandmother a nod, and left to attend to his business.

Grandfather helped his other half inside their home and put her at her favorite place to sit. Grandfather gave her a strong soup made from the roots of a healing plant readily available in their area.

It was not long before Grandmother was back on her feet and the two of them were discussing the situation. Of course, Grandmother was not a happy camper at this point. No matter how hard an effort she made, it seemed that the gathering of a totem medicine animal was not to be hers.

Now, this is a short version of an epic story. It takes a weekend or more to tell these kinds of stories that give our society guidelines on how to be right and to do good. We gather around and listen to the storyteller, taking breaks for lunch and dinner. After dinner, the epic story continues by campfire light…

Grandmother made many more attempts at her quest to gather a medicine animal, but all her attempts ended in failure.

One day word came that in a village far away a young maiden had been possessed by a demon spirit. All who had any wherewithal had already had a go at chasing this bad spirit from the maiden's body, but none had succeeded.

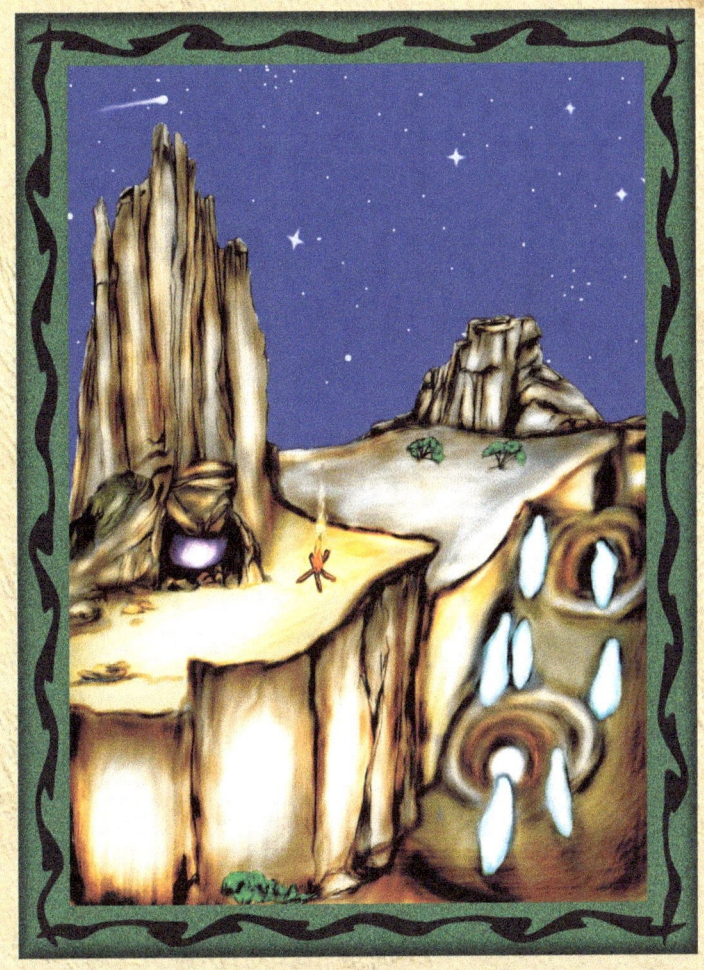

Mystery

When the long white-haired Grandmother heard about this, she decided to go to this young maiden and fix her up. As she went along barefooted, she gathered special plants, roots, leaves and skins, since she had learned a thing or two while walking the medicine wheel of life for so long. As she drew closer, news went out that a long white-haired Grandmother was coming from far away to exorcise the demon spirit inside the unfortunate individual.

When Grandmother got to the outer limits of the small village, a bunch of people gawked and stared at her. With closed hands over their mouths, they whispered low enough so Grandmother could not hear what they were saying. She knew something was up but had no idea what.

As she got close to the place where the young maiden lived, so many people were gathered there it seemed as if the whole village had accumulated in this one place.

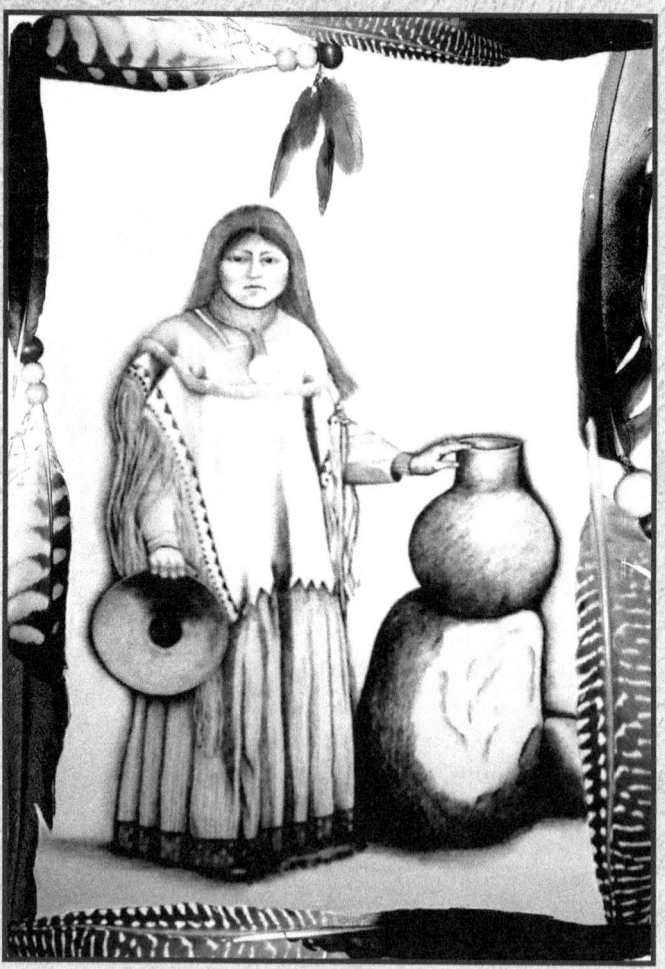

Apache Woman

The crowd parted for the old Grandmother and she was feeling uneasy. She came to do some healing work, yet she could not get a totem medicine animal to share knowledge of their healing attributes with her. She was really in a fix.

When Grandmother reached the door, she smelled a very foul odor coming from within and when she saw the young maiden, Grandmother just about fainted. The maiden was levitating in the air, her arms and legs bound by rope, attached to four stakes in the ground. Her chin resembled that of a

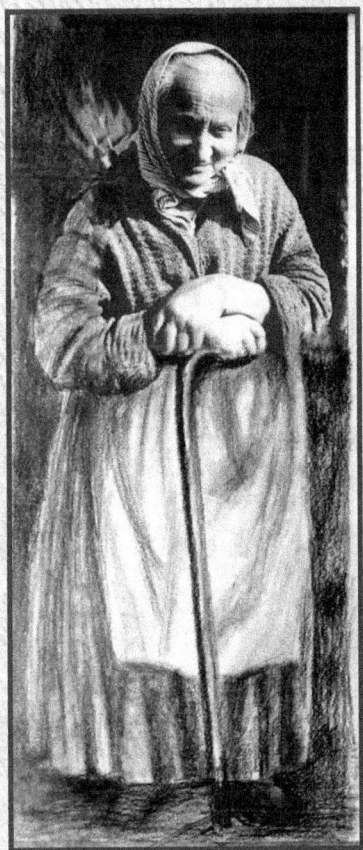

Babushka

frog's with its throat extended. Her chin had blown up like a balloon. She was speaking in a strange language no one had ever heard before and she was spitting foul globs from time to time. All the inner-circle people[7] were in the small home and they looked upon Grandmother as the last remaining hope for this disfavored youth.

Grandmother appeared confident, but inside she was asking herself, "What shall I do?" So she did some things that came naturally, like lighting on fire some dried plants she had gathered along the way and using the smoke to purify herself and the place where the healing was expected to happen. She also made tea from some roots and

---

[7] The inner-circle are those who come first and stay last.

added a few leaves of various sorts in an attempt to, at least, do something.

The maiden would not drink the herbal medicine tea, nothing was working, and the people were beginning to doubt the white-haired Grandmother. With everyone watching her every move, the pressure was on, and she was getting nowhere.

Realizing she had exhausted all her efforts and had no medicine to use, Grandmother stubbornly folded her arms and said out loud, "I will hold my breath until the demon spirit is driven out of this young maiden, or I will die right here." She was true to her word and began to get wobbly on her feet. She became dizzy and was just about to hit the floor when, to everyone's surprise, this little old Grandmother let out the biggest, loudest and stinkiest fart[8] imaginable. So foul was the stench that everyone fled the room, including the demon spirit.

The maiden hit the ground flat on her back[9], the wind knocked out of her. Slowly, she began to regain consciousness. She cried and thanked Grandmother many times for what had been done.

This is the end of the story. In Native American cultures, the stories are not 'summed up' for the listener. They are told this way so that anyone who hears them may draw a different conclusion as to what happened and what it means. This way, your own individual medicine comes into play so you can understand them for yourself.

All things in their own time.

---

[8] Also known as flatulence, barking spider, air biscuit, and ou toot, a bad-smelling gas that comes from between your legs.
[9] Exorcisms are a dangerous thing to deal with and can have very serious consequences. So please do yourself and your family a big favor and leave this to those with experience in such matters.

WESTERN PRAYER VS. INDIGENOUS PRAYER

In dealing with prayer, conceptually speaking, methodology is important. If someone has a broken arm, the usual prayer might go something like this: "Creator (or whomever you pray to[10]), fix my broken arm." In this way, it is very powerfully put out into the "Great Mystery" and now has the opportunity to actually manifest[11]. However there are even more powerful ways of accomplishing the task at hand.

Indigenous types of prayer, whether they are Native American, Japanese, Korean, or Chinese, share a commonality: they are conceptual as opposed to literal. Spirituality is the way of the indigenous people of the world. It has its origins in time immortal. The concept of prayer is different than the Western dogma that has been relatively new for Two Leggeds[12]. I predict that spirituality based on one almighty "Creator" is the way things shall return to, with the heart as your guide as opposed to books of rules. In the spiritual aspect, books of rules are not needed because everyone has a heart.

As we grow up, our school systems tend to our minds and bodies, preparing us as our governments see fit to turn us into "contributing members of society." But as Two Leggeds, we are not just a mind and a body. What about our spiritual needs?

Some people adopt the spiritual practices of their parents simply because that is what they were exposed to. Is it the best choice for them individually? This series of books are available to those seeking alternative ways.

---

[10] In doubt whom to pray to? Imagine you're on a plane, the pilot says, "I have good news and bad news. Bad news is we're going to crash. Good news is you have 5 minutes to make your peace." Whomever you speak to in those five minutes is the answer to your question.

[11] As it is above so it is below.

[12] Native American people in many tribes recognize people by the number of legs they have, i.e. a one legged person is a tree, many legged is an insect person, etc.

So take a family whose father is successful, has made it through great difficulty, rising in his field of expertise. Perhaps he has had to step on others to get to a higher level. Then, when he throws a party, people only come if they think they will gain something from him in the process. He finds he has no friends. So he seeks to fill the void he knows is there. But what is it? How did it get there and what is the craving to now know?

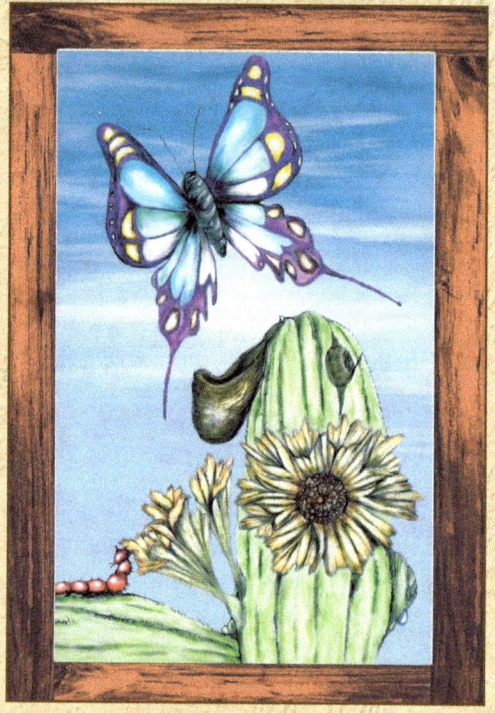

Transformation

This tends to be a lack of ceremony; a lack of spirituality that he may not even know he is missing. This series of books is designed to bring spirituality to the forefront of thought and activity, to assist those in re-remembering that which they may have put aside for some time, an alternative.

SPIRITUAL WARRIORS

Prayer is one of the most valuable tools of spiritual warfare in our arsenal as Spiritual Warriors.

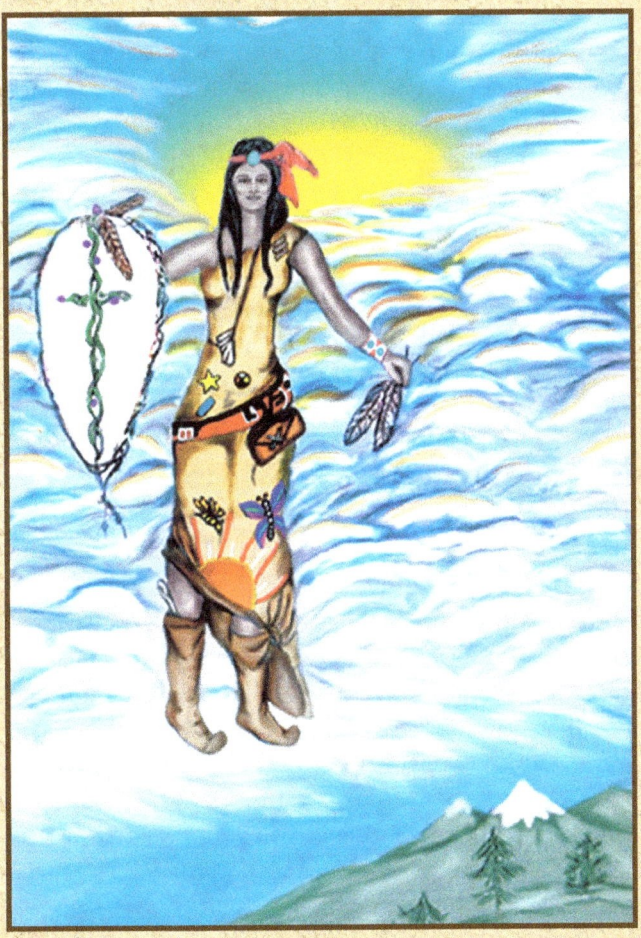

Spiritual Warrior

Spiritual Warriors are the ones represented by the horseshoe. The horse symbolizes the one who carries the burden of the people, and as Spiritual Warriors we carry the burden of the people willingly, on our shoulders.

Some examples of Spiritual Warriors: the ones who stand in front of tree cutters or even sit in trees to prevent the trees from being killed; the ones who will do something in relation to polluters who work with maliciousness towards our Mother Earth. Don't they see their grandchildren?

In traveling the world as a healer, many of spiritual warriors have been trained. The best venue has been the Boy Scout Camps, because it is easy to sit down with a large group and teach them all at the same time. The three-day training camp usually has a Sweat Lodge[13] on Saturday and teaching for the rest of the weekend.

Upon completion of these teachings, they emerge as fully trained and equipped Rainbow Warriors, so called because they come in many colors, shapes and sizes.

As it is told in the indigenous prophesies of Turtle Island, the next significant battlefield is in the spiritual arena. The dark side is gathering their forces and so, too, must we in the light gather our warriors for the good of all. It is not so easy to be a warrior of this calibre, but it is possible and makes no difference if you are female, male, young, old, handicapped, or have mental or physical challenges of any kind. One must be strong inside and have a determination and commitment to be right, to do right and to be brave.

One time while at a lecture in Austin, Texas in the 1990's, a Grandmother stood and said, "Thank you, Two Feather. It only takes one warrior to stand-up and be heard."

Round and round the polluting smokestack, we dance for our mother ~ Earth.

---

[13] See "Sacred Ceremonies" later in this book for a description of this ceremony.

PRAYER IS NOT JUST ASKING

Prayer is an expansion of oneself to join with the Great Spirit (or whatever you call this being: Creator, God, Buddha, etc.) to be at one, connected with the soul of life.

Prayer is not only a place to go in times of need, but also a place to rejoice and be thankful in times of plenty, in truth and in fullness.

As with Animal Medicine, you can learn to be more attuned to energies everywhere around you that can assist in prayer. If you live amongst the mountains, you can understand the medicine there. If you live near the sea, you can be attuned to the mystery, magic, and energy of the ocean. These are not imagined things; they are forces as real as you or me, and every bit as big as the three dimensional world we live in, yet so pure. All a part of the whole, "All My Relations."

Prayer is a merging of ourselves; a time when we remove ourselves from the solidity of being 'only one' of this Earth and put ourselves out there amongst unseen forces, which are part of what makes up our world. In faith, we accept that we are not alone, that we are the world and the world is us. It is good to re-remember that you have the power within you. It is time to create a link between the old ways and the new, to keep true conceptual prayer animate in our modern world.

Let us keep the light of our ancestors with us and keep the circle alive[14]. Pray in a good way and with a good heart, and, in so doing, harm no one or no thing.

---

[14] This is a battle cry for light warriors to recall where we came from and to recall those who made the ultimate sacrifice so we could be free today.

When praying be aware of what you ask for. Ensure it is coming from a good heart, hurts no one and no thing, and is done in a good way; then you can feel confident that whatever comes to pass has the potential of being as a direct result of the intention of your prayer.

RHYME WITH NO RHYME

Round and round we go into their dreams
Round and round we remind them,
of their sons and daughters

Round and round they will drink the same
water and eat the same food as the rest of us
Round and round we dance whence we
come we'll be sure we don't go again

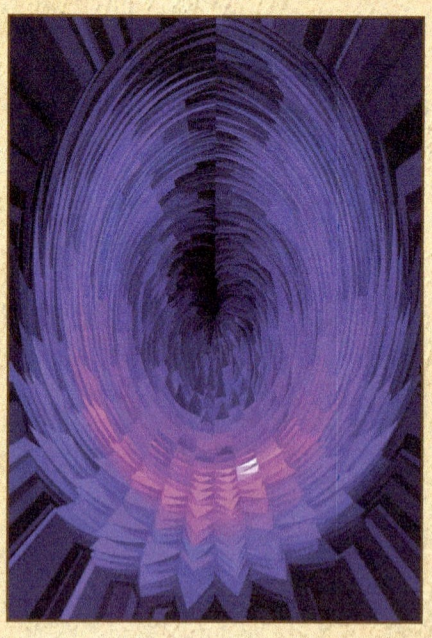

MONEY AND MATERIAL ITEMS

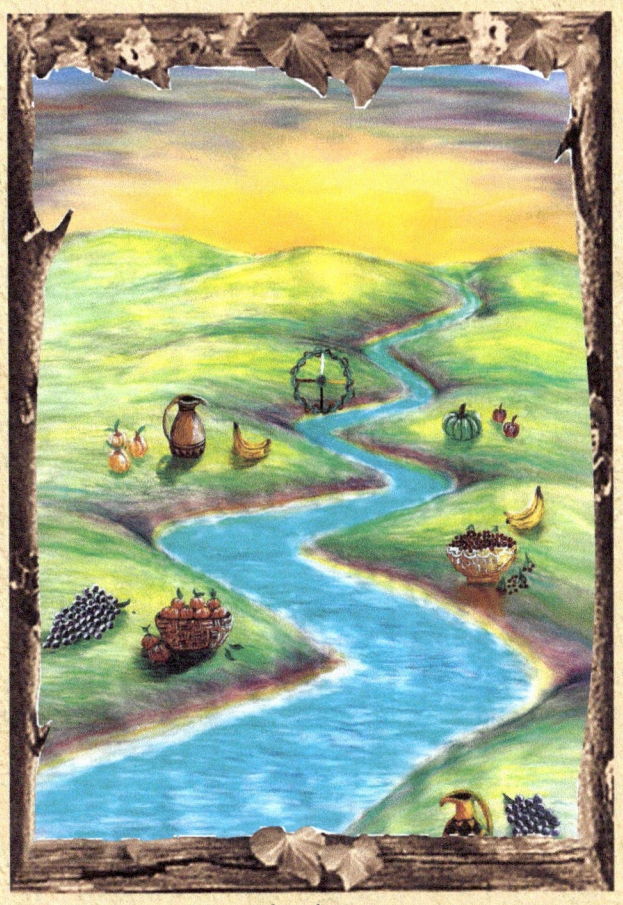

Abundance

Some have ideas about money and material items in relation to prayer which come from a place of obscurity and preconceived notions. When people come to me with issues in the area of finances, and ask "Two Feather, I am in financial difficulty. My family is suffering but it just doesn't seem right to pray for money and I don't know what to do." I reply by saying, "If someone were sick in your family, you would pray for them, wouldn't you? Wouldn't you pray for the trees in the

Amazon, if they were being killed in mass quantities? If the object of your prayers was someone of another race, wouldn't you pray for them, also? If something was terribly wrong, wouldn't you ask Creator or Spirit to return it to balance? Then why not pray for money when it is needed?

If your car needs replacing and you just lost your job and your family and associates are depending on you financially and you need $3,000 to get another vehicle or to have another shot at a job, then go ahead and ask for $3,000.

Since some people have difficulty giving themselves permission to pray for money, allow me: "I, William Two Feather, as a trained and initiated spiritual advisor, hereby give all seekers the permission and authority to pray for what you need," as opposed to what you want, in a good way and with a good heart.

You may pray for money, you may pray for material goods, but you should be careful what you ask for. A rule of thumb here is that if you want to pray for something in particular, but you are having doubts that it's coming from a good heart in a good way, then don't pray for it! Doubt can be a good measure of your inner truth.

"I can't pray for money" is a common theme. Indeed, this is a "grey area," to say the least. Clarity can be achieved in its own time, the time when it's appropriate to realize balance as part of the "natural order of the universe."

In this light, if you choose to seek the Native American way, here is how you could go about it. We believe special gifts can be found in each direction. [15]For material items, praying should be done facing the West. The West is the place of

---

[15] Whenever directions are referred to, it means the four directions: East, South, West, North, in that order. In many tribes, we believe that this is the natural flow of the universe, clockwise.

bountiful harvest. The seeds we planted in the East, the place of new beginnings those we then nurtured and protected as they grew in the South, are now ready to be reaped in the West. The color that represents the West is black (such as black clothing, jewelry, etc.), and the stone of power is obsidian. Some of my very own financial prayers[16] were answered minus $4.00. This was viewed as a spiritual charge, one for each of the directions – East, South, West and North.

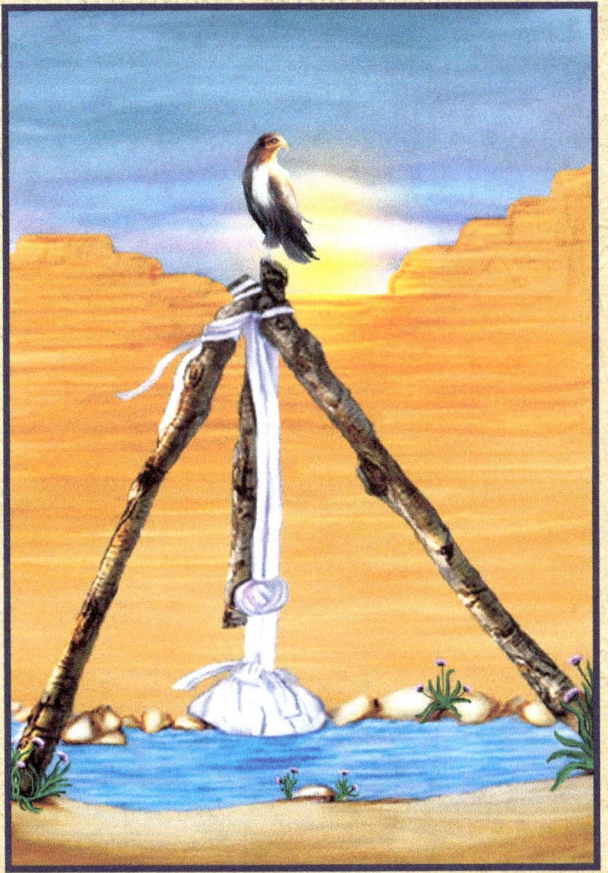

Weather Rock

---

[16] I can count the times prayer has been given for money on one hand, two times. This is done rarely, saving it for the times when really needed. That way it is easier to avoid abuse of prayer.

Story ~ Finances

In 2000 or 2001, I was in Albuquerque, New Mexico at the largest Pow Wow in the world, called Gathering of Nations.[17] For the sixth year in a row, we (N.A.S.P.) had a booth there selling Native American hand-held drums, flutes, CD's of my music[18] and other items. At the same time, my Harley Davidson motorcycle, called "Wind", was in the repair shop and I needed $2,200 to repair it. Now, this was prime riding season in New Mexico (USA) and Wind was (as if) my pony.

Pow Wow had begun, the prayer was for enough frog skins (USD) to get my pony outta mechanic's jail. The show was ending, however the goal was not met yet. Almost at the last minute, a woman came up to my booth and purchased the last of its kind Pow Wow drum called "The Rainbringer" for $600. Overall, the sum total of that weekend was $2196.00, enough to get Wind, the name of my Harley Davidson, all fixed up.

Be grateful and be sure to say "Thank You" to complete the circle. Be sure not to treat this as a menial activity. Menial activities are not conducive to constructive spiritual growth.

People ask me, "Two Feather, what if I want $2 million?" I ask, "Do you need $2 million?" They reply, "No, but I want $2 million." I ask, "Well, what do you need?" They reply, "Well, I really need about $200,000."

No one can stop them from praying for $2 million. However, remember to be careful for what you pray for, as this is a spiritual activity, and thus carries with it all that is

---

[17] About 50,000 tickets are sold every year to this great event. If you only go to one Pow Wow in your life, make it this one. You can find out more at www. gatheringofnations.com. This event has been known to sell out, so be sure to get tickets as soon as you've made the decision to go.
[18] Currently N.A.S.P..... (Native American Spiritual Prod.) has released 5 books of 12. The six indigenous flute music titles are "Indigenous Trance Dance", "Red Earth Danz", "Spiritual Warrior", "Unity Dance", "Red Medicine Dance", and "Elements." All can be found at the website: www.2feather.com.

representative of such functions. It may happen that your mother then dies in an accident and has an insurance policy for $2 million. You will get the $2 million you prayed for, your entire family will be missing mother, and after you have spent all the money, your mother will still be gone.

This is not a good thing. This is disrespect and abuse of medicine and prayer, which always has harsh ramifications. There is no escape from this.

Abuse of Medicine

Beware. If you abuse medicine in the spiritual realm, there is a much higher price to pay than in the non-spiritual realm. Here on this physical plane, you pay your little bit of money to the officials and you get your little piece of paper stamped and that's that.

But in the spiritual realm, it is not that easy, though, in essence, it is much simpler.

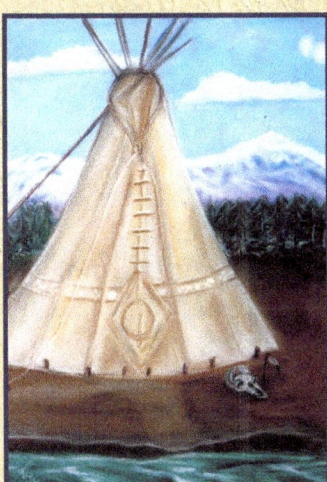

Tee Pee

MEDICINE OF ANIMALS

Some writers simply research other people's work, compile the information into a book and then present themselves as authorities on the subject. However, I believe that if one is to write about a teaching, one should have some hands-on experience.

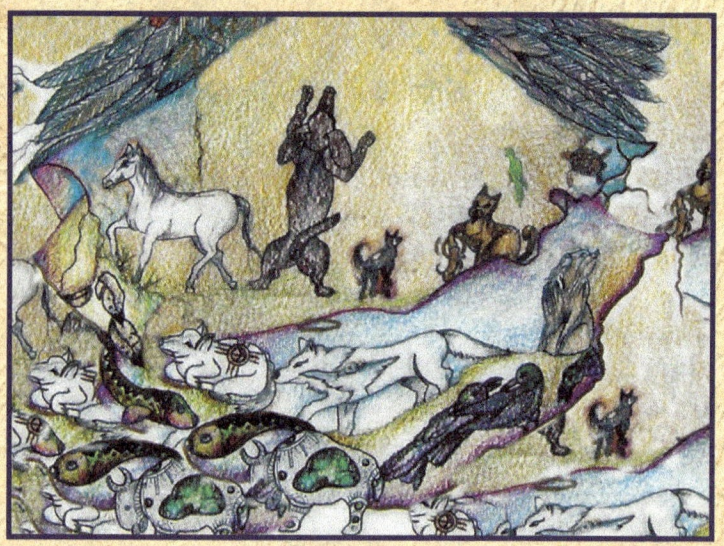

Animal Medicine

The teachings being presented here about Totem Medicine Animals, as well as all the teachings in this book and in the books in this series, come directly from my teachers, myself, and other genuine sources. It is my belief that first-hand teachings can more powerfully serve seekers on their path to spirituality, as well as helping them to understand the connection that their existence has to all their relations.

When it comes to animals and their medicine, one is advised to keep in mind that there are over 500 tribes on Turtle Island. In the West, their beliefs vary quite a bit from the East, which varies from the Northwest and the Southwest, which varies from the Dakotas, etc. The one concept that all tribes share is that, according to their species, all animals are endowed with particular attributes commonly referred to as "medicine."

To understand these medicines is to get a glimpse of how indigenous people have preserved many teachings. They are written here now for all people. Keep an open mind as some of these concepts may be different from the teachings you already have.

In the Native American world, there are twelve different kinds of people (or archetypes.) This is our equivalent of astrology, though our teachings are Earth-based, rather than star -based.

There are twelve totem animals; the particular attributes they are endowed with are commonly referred to as their "medicine." At birth, everyone is given a Totem Medicine Animal depending on the season under which they are born. This animal remains with them for their entire walk upon Earth Mother.

In a loose sense, one's totem animal depicts and determines the type of person they will be, since every person has special gifts related to their totem animal. Each animal also has a particular medicine color associated with him or her. When the person wears that color, it increases their gifts many-fold. All twelve totems have a stone of power, too.

How much a person actually avails themselves of these special gifts from Creator is a matter of individual choice, more or less. If you come to understand the medicine of these animals, many teachings can follow. Concerning yourself, it can help you to better understand your own medicine. Concerning others, it can help you to deal with them in ways appropriate to their medicine.

For example, Raven people are gullible and will believe almost anything you tell them, whereas Cougar people are naturally cautious, not wanting to reveal themselves; you'll have to prove yourself to cougars before they'll open up to you.

In the area of prayer, you can draw on the attributes of the totem animal you are in need of. For example, let us say you need to make something look beautiful and you're not really sure how to do it. The medicine of the Deer is to bring beauty to the world. If you call in Deer medicine to assist you, it can give you many new ideas about how to make your project beautiful. You can use will, manifestation and imagination.

If something needs to be done perfectly, you could call in Snow Goose medicine. They do not let anything get past them because they are perfectionists.

If you want to figure out how to help poor people, call in Elk medicine. The Elk has a strong sense of right and wrong and can help you figure out how to help people who cannot help themselves.

If you know you are going into a fight, you will want warrior energy so you call in Cougar medicine. They do not give up and they are unpredictable. Therefore, when you are fighting and the enemy is trying to figure out your next move, you will keep surprising them because you will be unpredictable.

If something is going on with you that you cannot figure out, you could call in the "looks-with-in" medicine of the Bear for some introspective answers.

In addition to the twelve medicine animals, I will bring in some other animals and their medicine. Observing these animals in the wild, undisturbed, can link us to these teachings from long ago.

When you understand medicine animals, you will have the

power, authority and dominion to build a solid foundation upon which to make decisions about the issues you face.

In the following section and throughout this book, animals may be referred to as 'she', 'he', 'Mr.' or 'Mrs.'; however, totem medicine animals are not gender specific. Whether male or female, an Otter has "peacekeeper" medicine. Likewise, whether male or female, a person born between January 20th and February 18th will have the Otter as their totem medicine animal.

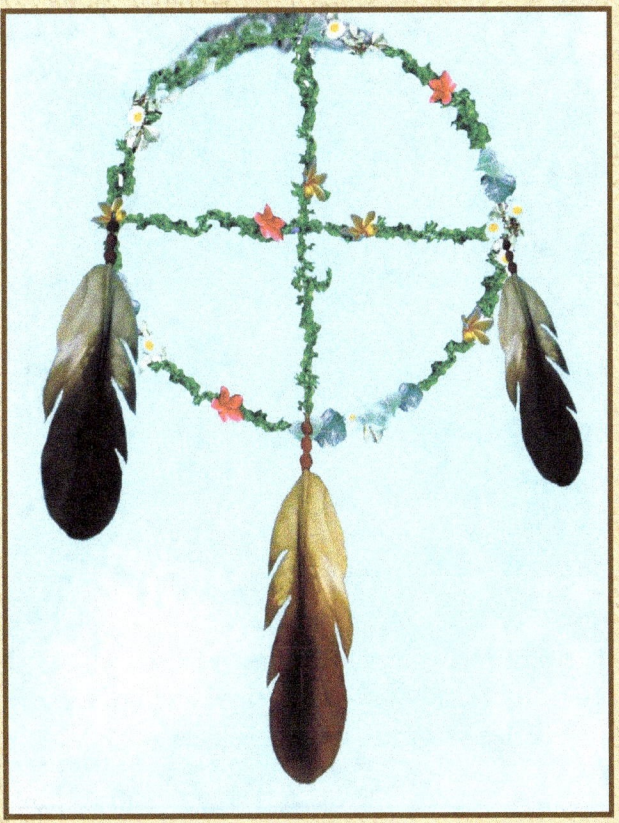

Medicine Wheel

Otter
Totem Animal if born January 20 - February 18
There are two varieties of otters: the river otter and the sea

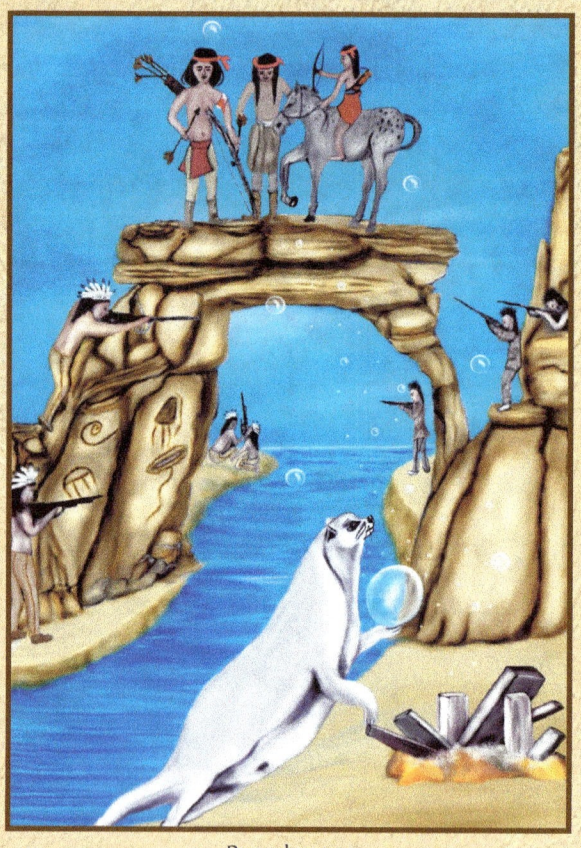

Peacekeeper

otter. They are quite different! These teachings refer to the river otter. Otter fur is very fine so they tend to it much, as in giving a lot of attention to personal hygiene.

The medicine of otters is "the peacekeeper." In the infinite wisdom of Creator, it was seen to it that the otter knows what two opposing sides are willing to accept. Say there is a labour dispute in a foreign land within some multi-national company. The boss, a self-made millionaire, sees that negotiations have broken down to a point where he needs to intervene personally. He goes to the bargaining table and brings his trusted advisor, a Beaver person. Since the boss is self-made, he believes he can smooth over the situation. However, he is doomed to failure. Even though his Beaver person is present giving sound council, the boss does it his own way and inevitably fails. If he were just a bit smarter, he would have brought in the Otter person to defuse the situation. They are fun loving and, in fact, must have fun or face the consequences.

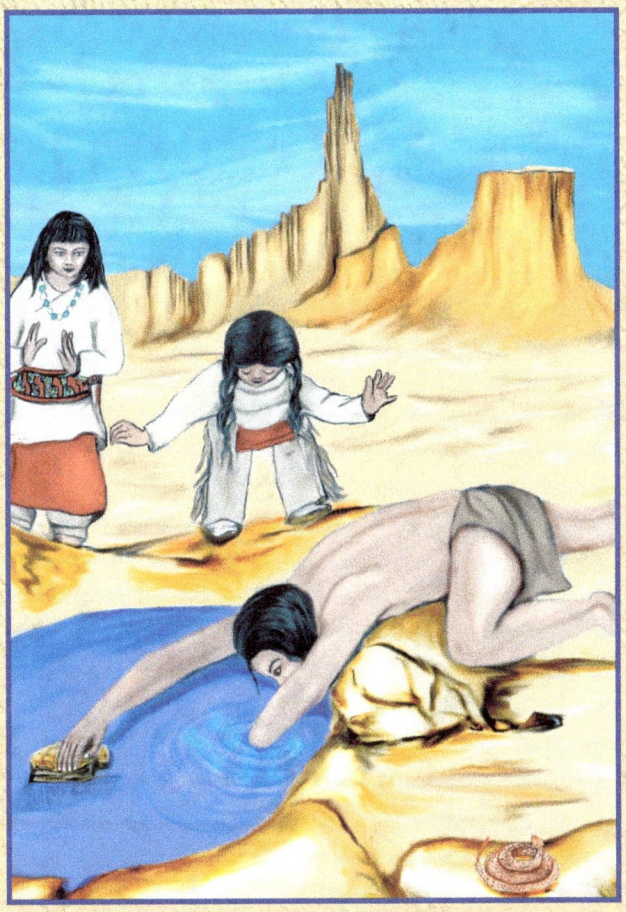

Innocence

When Otter gets sick, this usually manifests first in the form of constipation. This is easily remedied by going out and having fun. The Otter is always invited to most social gatherings; they are loved by all and inspire others to initiate fun activities, or initiate them themselves.

It is not good to put an Otter person in a small enclosed room and expect them to do well. They need to be active, sharing their special gift from Creator with others. In the final analysis, this is what this is all about, using your special gifts in the service of others and a clear understanding.

When it is your time to go to the next world, you will find a book there that shows you the life you have led on Mother Earth. This book will show such things as how you used your special gifts in the service of others. It is not a judgmental look so much as an informative perspective. Before you see this book, you must go past the hospital monitors that say flat line. In past some times when I was on this long journey that seemed short, that is where a person is near a table and that is where the book is.

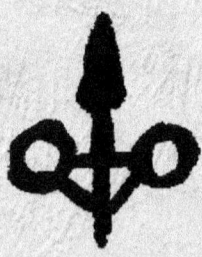

Cougar
Totem Animal if born February 19 - March 20

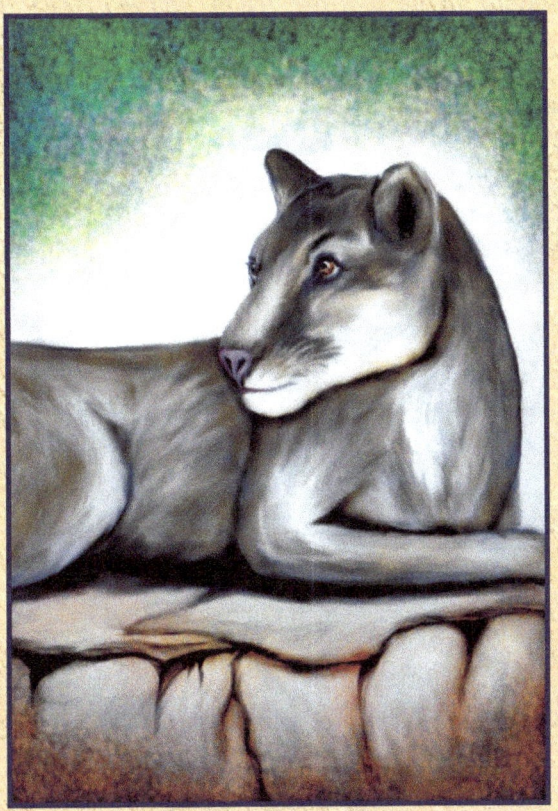

Cougar

Aka Mountain Lion. The medicine is that of "unpredictability." Might as well forget figuring cougars out; as soon as you think their strategy is visible, you are proved incorrect. Bravery and caution describe the cougar well.

He is wary of most things. In order for him to accept something, it needs to be proven or established somehow to his strictest satisfaction, before he will reveal himself.

I've been afforded the great privilege to work with youth[19] in trouble with the law on numerous occasions. In so doing, it is easy to see the people who are of cougar medicine.

When I arrive, all the counsellors come to greet me with extended hands in friendship and mutual respect; except one or two who stand in the background, visible and present, but strategically placed with their backs to some wall protection or cover. They usually have their arms folded and doubting chins tucked in, speaking in body language that signifies their caution. They invariably come to shake my hand, but only after they have seen that the Native American-based techniques have helped the youth in their charge to build self-esteem.

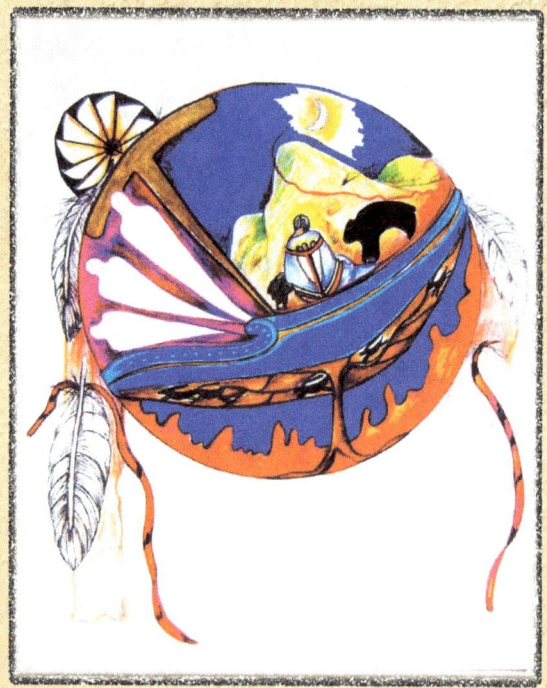

Medicine Shield

[19] *These abused and troubled youth have been through the fire and survived where most have perished. Some as young as 9 years old have killed several people, been arsonists or gang members, and have been molested from a young age.*

Red Tail Hawk
Totem Animal if born March 21 - April 19

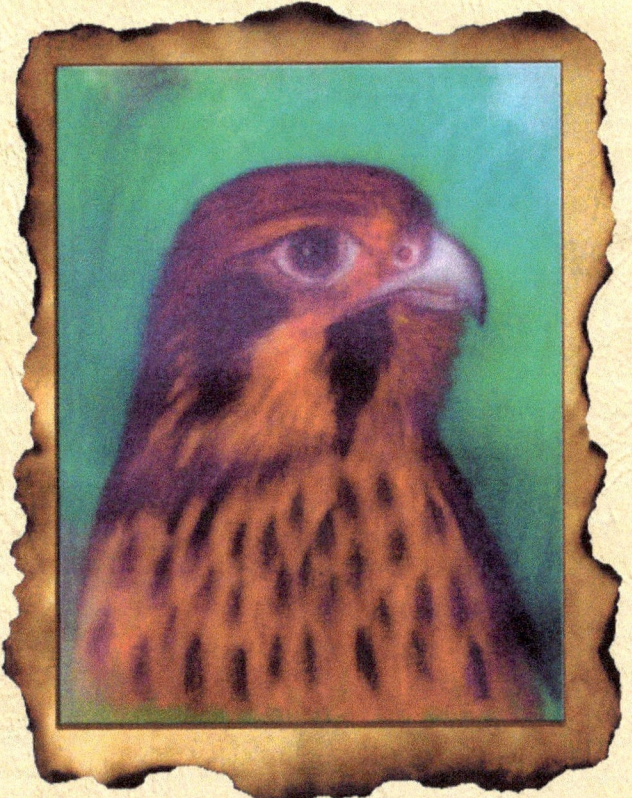

Red Tail Hawk

This bird of prey includes other varieties of hawks as well, the red tail being the epitome of hawk medicine. The medicine is "leadership, action and invention." The hawk is quick to fly into things and quick to fly out. While the wolf will sit around and savour his accomplishments, the hawk does not have time for such things; she's flying off to the next thing to do. The one word best applied is initiator.

Hawks have "far vision", which doesn't mean that they can see into the future so much as that they have an affinity for considering the consequences of their actions now and how it will effect the future in a week, a year, a lifetime, or three generations from now. However, they are not necessarily good at finishing things[20].

So let's say a group of 30 people who don't know each other have come together to do some task. They're milling around, unsure of what to do. The hawk is the one who stands up and says, "Alright, everyone, let's form an orderly line over here. We will start this task in the East and continue on until it is completed." For a while, the hawk will contribute to this group effort but soon enough, without much to do, he will dismiss himself to go off and tend to another flock, so to speak.

The hawk is drawn to the color yellow, and to golden yellow in particular, which increases their medicine when worn in times of action and initiation. They also have a strong draw to the precious gemstones called fire opals. The botryoidal (shape of grapes on a vine) structure inside of the stone represents the strength and conviction of the hawk as a passionate doer. They have an innate sense of justice that others may not share. I am a hawk person.

---

[20] This is not to infer that hawks cannot finish things; they can and with a "bang." However, this means to say that their special gift from Creator is to be the match that starts the blaze that will become a roaring fire.

Beaver
Totem Animal if born April 20 - May 20

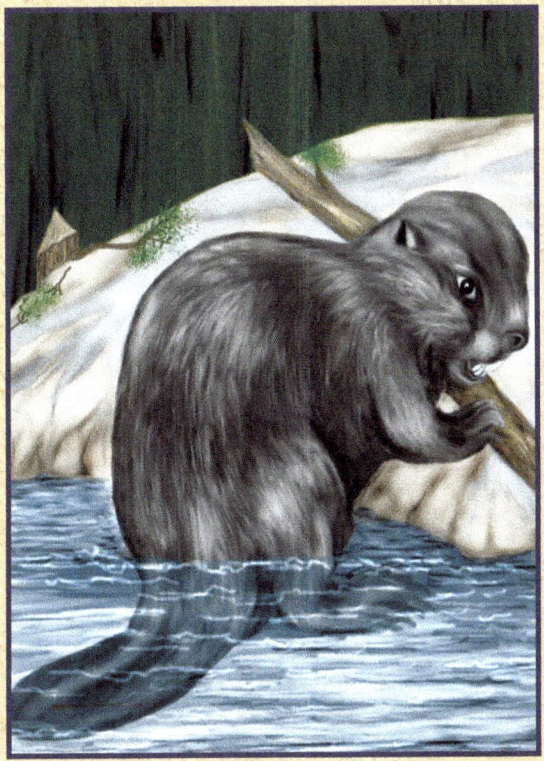

Beaver

The beaver family is hard working, always cutting down small trees, gathering food, and tending to the beaver family home. They are industrious and not ones to sit about idly. They sound an alarm to warn everyone before a tree is felled. They stay solitary, a complete unit; one beaver family to a pond is customary. And they like to be snug as a bug in a rug with their very soft full fur.

Beavers carry their tools with them: their two big front teeth are prominent. They keep things to themselves, and this keeping in of feelings is as effective as the dams they construct. The restriction of the river is synonymous with the flow of the river. Their favorite color is blue and they have an affinity for blue colored stones.

Beavers are constantly spiritually growing from a young age until the end of life as we know it. The Beaver person, much like the beaver, holds back their emotions like the dam of a river.

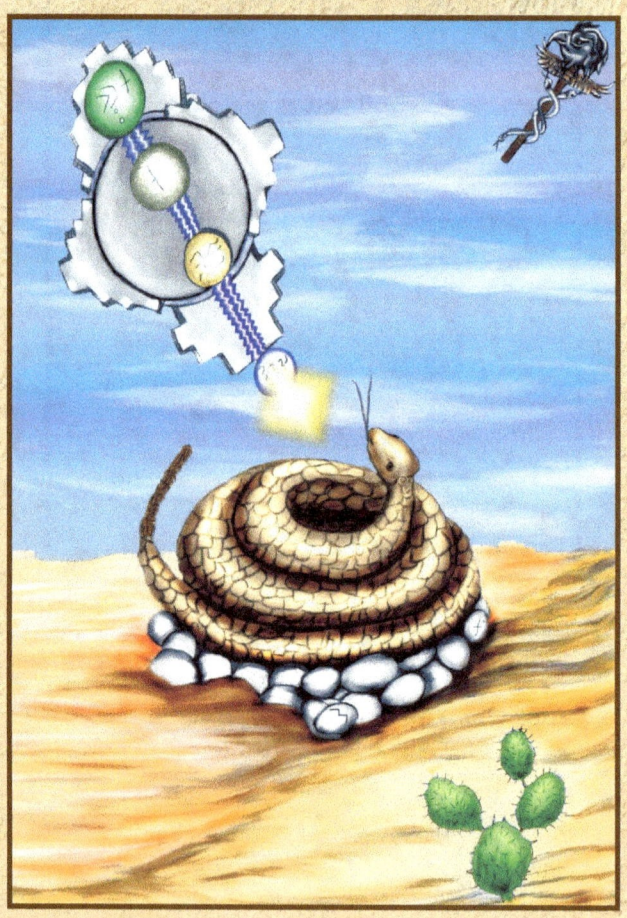

Healing

Deer
Totem Animal if born May 21 - June 20

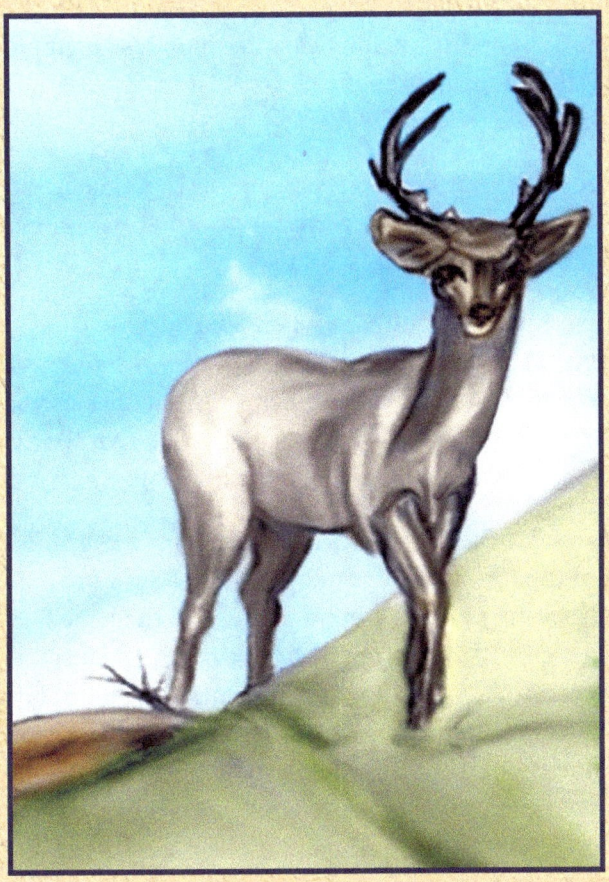

Deer

"The bringer of beauty" is the medicine of the Deer. They are creative and have a flair for art, decorating, and just making things look beautiful. Those who have no teachings of such things often misunderstand the 4-legged Deer People.

All people have some knowledge of self-healing as a part of homeostasis, the being-ness of sentience. So if a Bear person gets shot in the shoulder and needs to get healed, she would go up into the mountains to a place with five hot mud pools.

Now which one should she go into? She can only choose one, and all have different properties. The Bear chooses the one that will draw the bullet from her body, and she gets well. A dog gets a cut on his leg and licks the wound, knowing there is something special in his saliva to assist in sterilization and healing.

The Deer (the Four Legged People) know more medicine plants than all the other animals put together, except maybe the Two Leggeds (and this is a subjective call.)

In Native American cultures, when the young Two Leggeds are playing, the old Two Leggeds keep an eye on them to see what tendencies they display; it helps the old ones decide what training the young ones are best suited for so that they will grow to be contributing members of their community.

Here is a story that illustrates this. There was a baby bird that fell from the tree and the young Two Leggeds saw this and started kicking the bird around. But one of the little ones, a ten year old - girl, would not do such a thing; she just sat on the sidelines and waited for her opportunity. A loud sound occurred and the attention of the little ones was diverted for a moment, just long enough for her to run over and get the baby bird away from them before they noticed. Then she tied sinew and some sticks to the little bird's broken wing, in an attempt to bring some healing. Seeing her do this, the old ones, Grandmothers and Grandfathers, spoke amongst themselves. They decided that this young one would be considered for training as a healer for her people.

The medicine person was made aware of their decision and he agreed to test the young one to see if she had what it would most certainly take to be a healer. He notified her of her assignment: for 30 moons, she must follow the deer people to gain their knowledge of the One-Legged ones, the plant people. Then she was to return and show the medicine person what she had learned. The youth was given strict orders not to disturb the deer people, and to be respectful.

For a 10 years old this was quite a task. After all, who else follows the deer? The meat eaters, the predators, and sometimes in packs. With only nine years on her Earth walk, for this youth just to survive would be a task in itself, let alone for her to be able to learn from the deer people. Most of the time, the young ones who undertake this task never return home.

So, taking along only a few days supply of food, the young one left. She found the deer people and began to follow them from a distance, but when the deer tribe stopped to eat, all the deer people were eating a certain kind of grass, while one lone deer was eating the leaves from a tree. When the young apprentice-in-testing slowly and quietly approached this deer, she noticed that the deer had green stuff coming from his nose. Upon scrutiny, she saw there was also green goo coming from his mouth and eyes.

"Hmm," the young one said to herself, this "One-Legged's" leaves give medicine that is good for sick eyes, nose and mouth.

She collected some of the leaves. Right then and there, and for the duration of her adventure/test, she made an offering every time she gathered such medicines, always mindful to complete the circle and "keep the balance."

The Deer people moved on. One of them slipped and broke his leg. He did his best to keep up with the herd but soon fell behind. Eventually the herd stopped to eat. But when the wounded deer caught up to them, he went to a different bush from the one everyone else was eating. With his good hoof, he dug around the plant to expose the roots, and thoroughly rubbed his broken leg on the root of this special plant. The young girl saw this and gathered some of the root into her medicine bundle.

She continued this kind of following, observing and collecting until the 20 moons were up. Then she returned to the tribe and reported directly to the medicine person. She shared all she had learned on her adventure, opening up the bundle she had clenched for 30 moons, and saying excitedly, "Oh! This is for broken bones. This is for ailing eyes, ears and mouth," etc.

The medicine person then accepted this youth for teaching, and the family was very, very proud to let their daughter study with him. When I was in a Japanese school telling this story, one of the youth raised his hand and asked, "Mr. Two Feather, do Deer speak Japanese or do we have to speak Deer talk?"

What rewards come from doing such spiritual work!

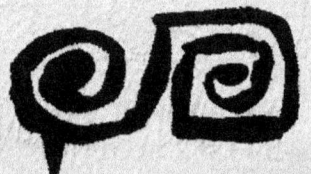

Swallow
Totem Animal if born June 21 - July 22

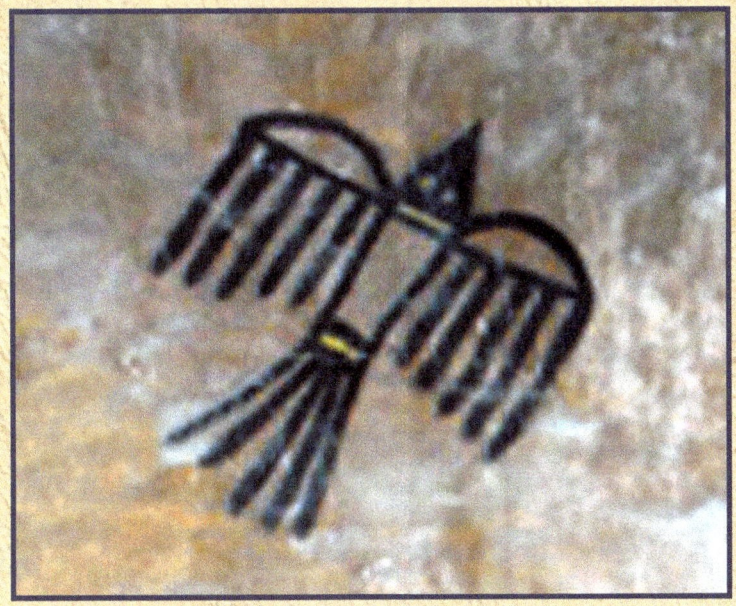

Swallow

This is the medicine I refer to as "chameleon medicine", the ability to get into and out of places easily.

With swallow medicine, it becomes easy to sit with generals and high-ranking officials tonight and enjoy a fancy meal using all the right forks and spoons, and then tomorrow, go sit with poor people and be equally accepted, having a meal served on plant leaves and eating with your fingers.

If a group is given the task of getting through a very dense forest in order to get to the other side of a mountain, swallow medicine will allow the shortest and best route to be figured out easily with the least amount of resistance. The swallow will be on the other side, looking down on everyone else and thinking to himself , "Look, right there is the best way to go," while pointing with his hand.

They reflect their environment easily and receptively. One pitfall is that the swallow can get so caught up in change and adapting that they can loose sight of themselves. It is advised to take care to embrace their own identity.

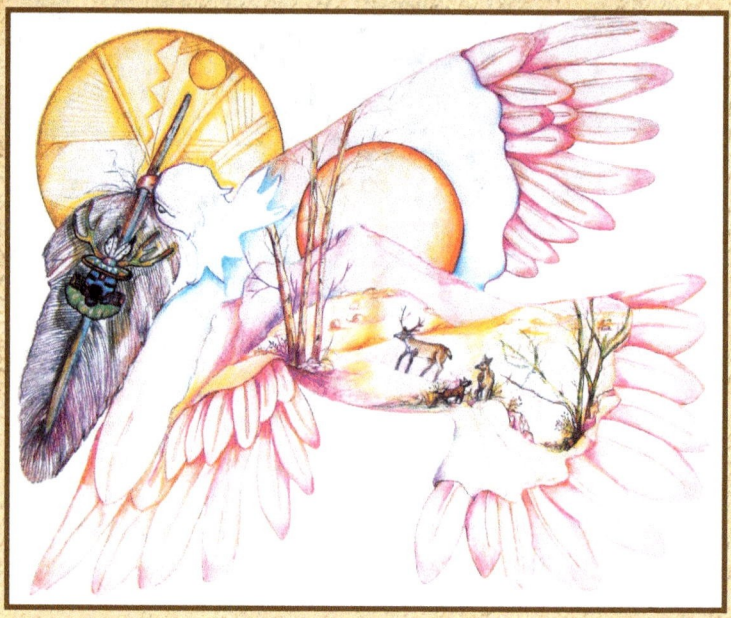

Peace Bird in Flight

They may ask "How do I get to me?" One suggestion is to go outside where it is not likely to be disturbed. Burn some white sage to get smoke. Put the smoke around you with moving hands. Then pray in your own way - asking spirits of "The Light" show me . . .

Sturgeon
Totem Animal if born July 23 - August 22

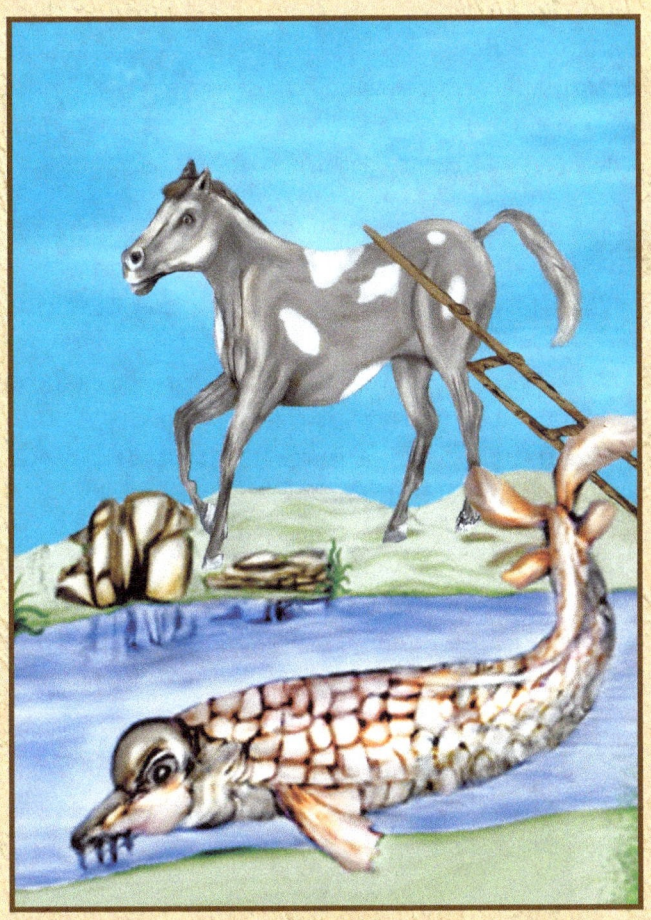

Sturgeon / Truth

This fresh water fish at the top of the food chain eats everything and nothing eats it[21]. There is strong armour on the outside of this fish; hitting him with a baseball bat with great force would not even inflict damage on his thick outer layer of protection.

---

[21] I concede that some people eat sturgeons and like grizzly bears, but let us not get caught up in particulars. It is my duty to share our ways and beliefs in the hope it may somehow benefit someone who cares to enrich themselves.

This fish favours the color red and has special medicine of "clear vision", the ability to see the truth. If someone lies to a Sturgeon, the fish will know by the second word out of the liar's mouth, if not sooner. The Sturgeon has great intuition in this particular area and should trust his first instincts, although he tends to over-intellectualize. If his hard armour is pierced, there is a treasure within.

So who would benefit from such medicine? A CPS[22] worker, for instance. What if a family is having serious problems and is brought before an official? All five family members have different stories. The official must make a critical decision. It might even mean breaking the family apart. That official has the right and authority to do so for the good of everyone concerned. If the official is a Sturgeon, he will be wise and will dole out justice swiftly and justly.

Sturgeons are sometimes seen as "know it all," and have a tendency to be argumentative. To be content with a partner, the Sturgeon requires someone who has strengths equal to his or hers. They may have difficulties in the area of relationships.

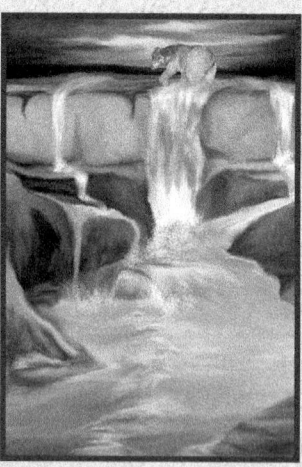

Bear in the water

---

[22] An acronym for a person who works for the child protection services.

Bear
Totem Animal if born August 23 - September 22

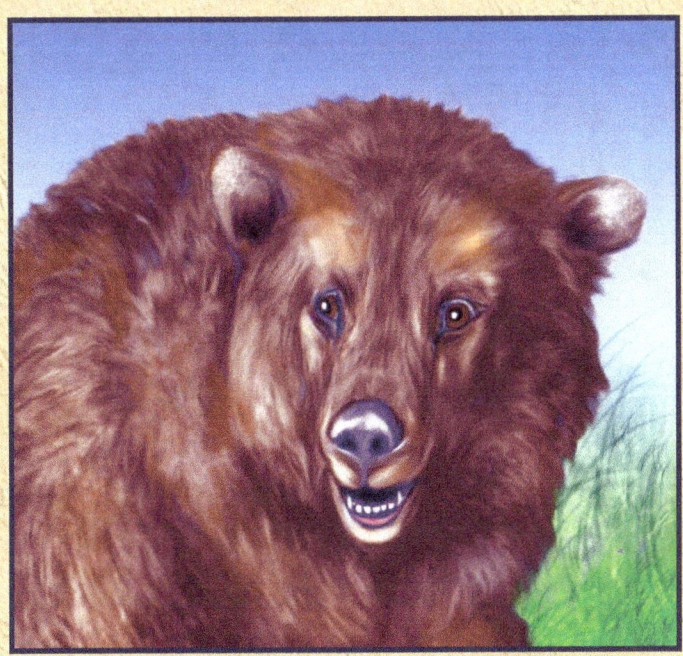

Bear

This is the medicine of the West, the place where the sun, after being carried in the talons of the Great Eagle, sets itself to rest. The medicine of the bear is that of introspection.

We refer to this medicine as "looks with-in" medicine. While in hibernation, the bear has much time with himself, and therefore has inner wisdom. Of all the animals, the bear ranks as one of the highest in this regard; however, bears tend to intellectualize instead of using their introspective medicine and have tendencies to circumvent their good fortune, which can lead to cheating themselves.

Mrs. Bear went to the store with $12 in her pocket to buy eggs, bread, and fruit; but her plan was to only spend $6. When she walked past the lottery machine, she had a feeling she knew the numbers. "Um, yes, let's see… 12… 16… 24… 36… 45, and the power number is 8." Then her head began to whirl with thoughts. "If I try the lottery, the odds are 26 million to 1. But if I spend the rest of the money on canned goods, my family will have food for a few more days." So she spent all $12 on food and went home.

The next day, Mrs. Bear happened to pass by the television just as the lucky lottery numbers were being called. Her jaw practically dropped to the ground as she heard her numbers announced one by one. "12-16-24-36-45." When the power number of 8 came up, she nearly fainted.

Some people assume that the bear charges into a fight, arms wildly swinging. In fact, the bear will first use his intuition to assess his enemy to determine their weakest spot; then the bear strikes once with accuracy, and it is all over.

The bear represents strength and purification, the "cleaner-upper", and tend to be grouchy. They love their home /cave, are basically antisocial and do not like outsiders on their turf. They are easily distinguishable by their walk—sombre, deliberate, mostly slow, and kind of mechanical in nature and gesture.

If we look at a match like a raven and bear, the bear wants to stay home and the raven wants to go out and be social. Most matchmakers will say this is a doomed relationship. I say not. If the bear likes to stay home, he will say, "Don't go," and the raven will say, "Don't stay home, go with me." But the bear usually will not and this could cause friction; but as long as everyone understands one another, there can be symbiosis. The loyal raven can go out, have some social activity, and then return home to the bear, an anchor that the lofty raven doesn't have much of. As for the homebody bear, he can live vicariously through the raven's tales of adventure. Therefore, each can be of benefit to the other.

Raven
Totem Animal if born September 23 - October 23

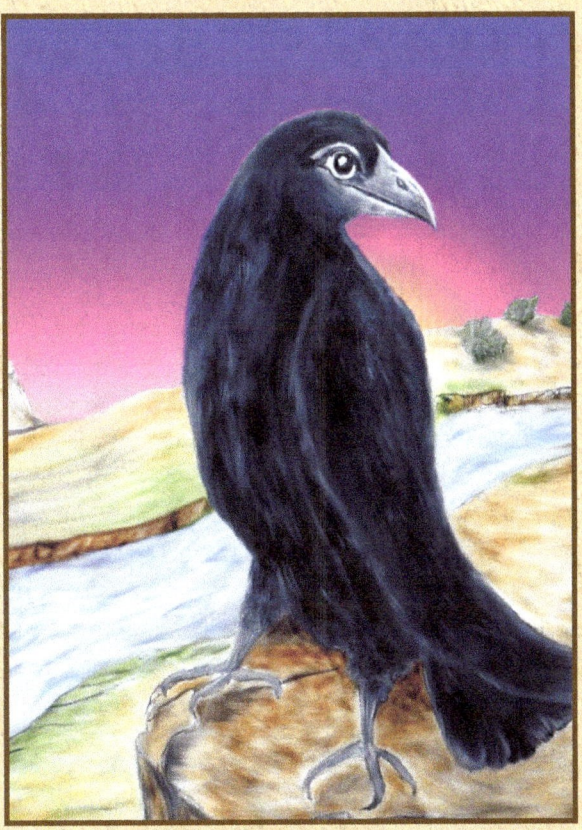

Ravens are not happy when they are called Crows.
That is why their name is Raven. The difference is that
one has a fan tail and one has a boxed tail.

This critter lives in many geographical areas, and although I am familiar with a few of them, I will address here the Native American Teachings.

This animal has the medicine of being able to transcend into spirit world, practically at the snap of the fingers. This is as great a medicine as there is among all of the Totem Medicine Animals. Imagine having the ability to go into the spirit world, even if for just a moment. The raven does this easily.

I participated in a Native American ceremony that entailed having my chest pierced with a tether that attached me to the tree of life. For four days I danced under a very hot sun, bare-chested and barefooted, with no food or water, in the hopes of going into spirit world to see what the course of my life would be for the next year, or for whatever time might be revealed to me. Deprivation of water, deprivation of sleep, deprivation of outside contact, etc. My point here is that if an animal is not your totem medicine animal, you can still avail yourself of their medicine; it will just take more effort.

One purpose the raven has to go into spirit world is to retrieve messages and bring them back for others, to assist them on their walk upon the medicine wheel of life. Most of the time ravens do not have to understand the messages they carry into this world, just deliver them. However, sometimes to the raven this can be overwhelming in that they feel they must know. But they do not know, and many of the messages only have significance to the receiver. It is not the place for ravens to interfere and ask the receiver, "What does that mean to you?" That is one place where ravens get themselves into trouble; they have been known to be meddlesome.

Ravens are very loyal, group-orientated animals and must have social interaction to remain healthy[23]. They flee at the first sign of danger and rightfully so, as Creator has given them this attribute as a means of survival. No worries: Cougar and Hawk, Wolverine and Elk will remain behind to fight. Ravens are not particularly liked amongst the rest of the animals, and are seldom invited for frivolities because they may start some trouble or turmoil. Ravens are dreamers, even if it is daydreaming, even if it is in school. They are the ones always looking out the windows while the teacher is giving the lessons.

---

[23] In Book of Spirit, Vol. 3, Doctoring, there is a real nice story of raven medicine and how it works.

Snake
Totem Animal if born October 24 - November 21

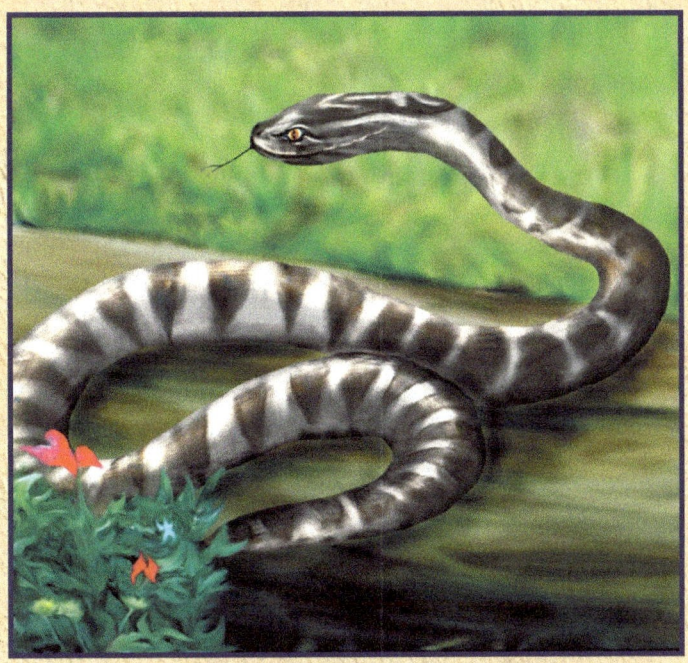

Snake

In most indigenous cultures I have been in contact with, the snake has a connotation of medicine and healing. The AMA uses two curled up snakes on a staff to represent their medical association.[24] The Ancient Egyptians saw the snake as having mystical properties, as did the indigenous people of Turtle Island.

A snake can come into a situation that has been functioning at the status quo for many years, and in a matter of just a few minutes, can rewrite the whole program and make the situation much more efficient.

Movers and shakers, snakes are swift to strike back when dealt

---

[24] *The symbol of the American Medical Association in the United States is a caduceus.*

with wrongly. When counselling a snake person, I ask them to please count to three before returning a strike, in an attempt to prevent more damage. With other totem animals, I would counsel them to count to ten; however, a snake does not have that kind of patience, so requesting such a long count would be sheer lunacy and tend to get no results at all.

Orange is the color of the snake. He has a vibrational frequency that increases the effectiveness of healing, as this is his medicine.

Snakes are suspicious. This is a survival tool given from Creator to snakes, so for them to give that away would be to give away the security of their own survival. It could be toned down a bit, though, as a snake's suspicion tends to keep them from learning important lessons of life.

It is possible to go against the nature of the medicine of the three snakes and 1 eagle head, as it is with all other medicines, but not advisable.

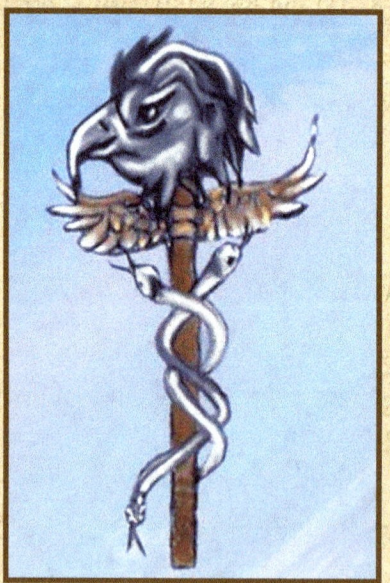

Skin Cadaceus

Elk
Totem Animal if born November 22 - December 21

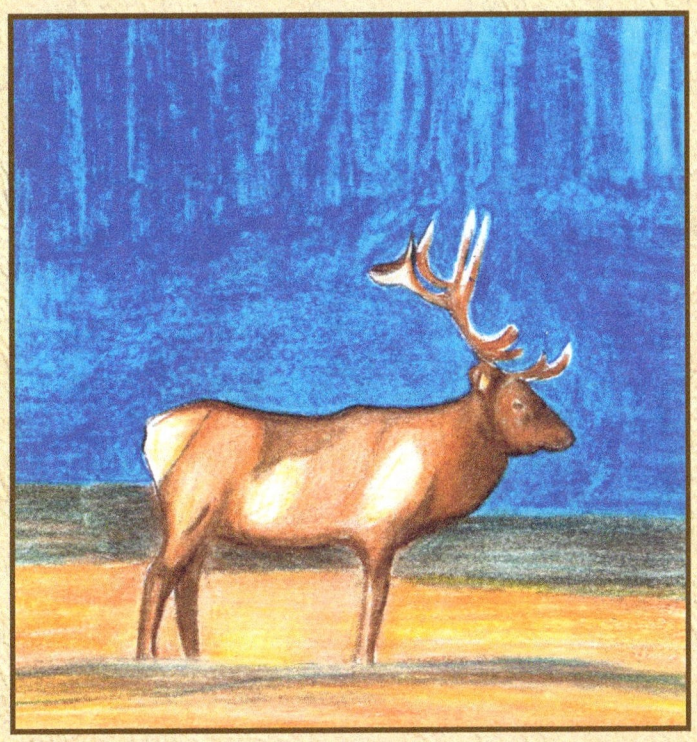

Elk

Looks like a very big deer but is not a deer; she is an Elk. They live in high places, and revel in high places, not only geographically speaking but in a life-sense.

If an Elk is working in a factory along with many other workers, she will not be satisfied with just a pay check at the end of the pay period. She is hard-working and always striving for the boss's chair. Rightfully so, the Elk is royalty in the kingdom of the animals. The Elk is the one who watches over all the others and who will trumpet loudly if any danger or injustice is about. When given authority, the Elk will use it to serve the people and not themselves. The elk is not inclined to have a self-serving mind-set. Elks are sought after for advice and they are adept at taking the regal way out. To be a high achiever takes a tough intense fortitude aka guts/bravery. They may not easily see that until confronted with challenges that will test this bravery.

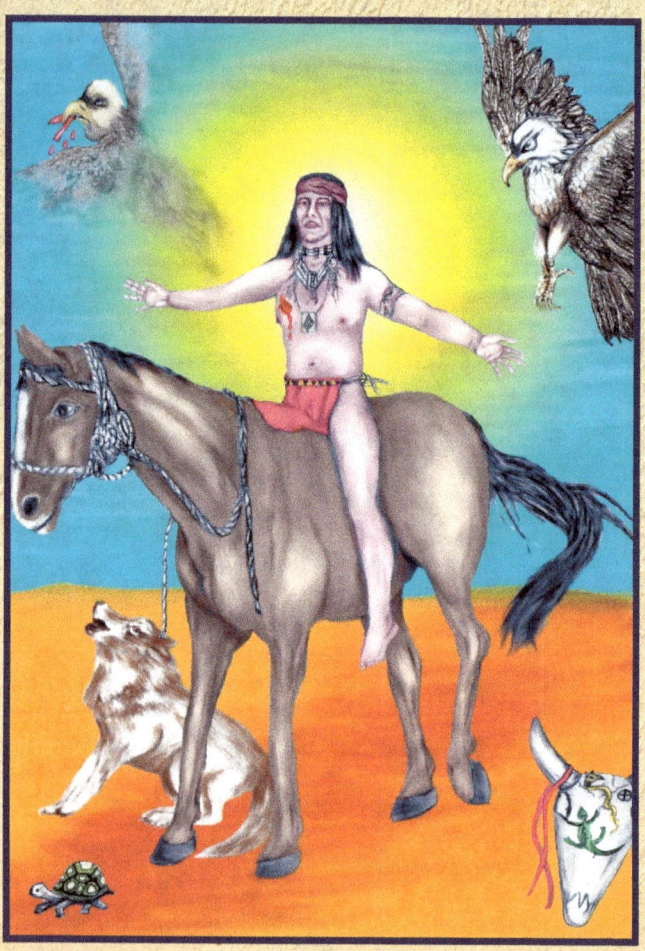

Initiation

Snow Goose
Totem Animal if born December 22 - January 19

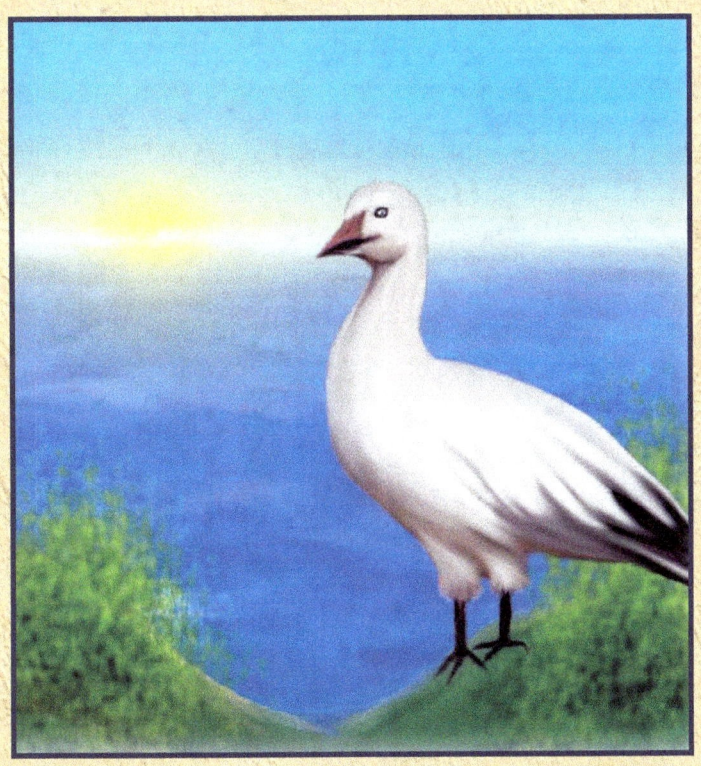

Snow Goose

The snow goose is the animal of the North, and "perfectionist" is the attribute. Snow geese respect and honor authority, and are very trustworthy. Being of the North puts them in a place of knowledge and wisdom, represented by the color white.

This is the time for snow, when Earth Mother provides her white blanket to most, giving medicine for rest and rejuvenation before the thawing snow and ice gives way to the newness and freshness of rebirth ~ Spring. Then the medicine wheel of life starts all over again. The cycle is the underlying principle of life and assistance so fundamental to Native American existence.

One year at Sundance[25], I heard the Elders tell this story (thank you): There was a multi-communal Indian function, and many of the ceremonial elders in attendance were of the Snow Goose Clan. One of the other guys, a big Indian, was talking loudly and being a bit obnoxious. He said, "Oh, I think I will go hunting and get me a goose for dinner." Just then, a flock of Snow Geese flew overhead. One big very wet, long, oozy glob of bird poop dropped down and landed right smack in someone's face. Guess who?

The Snow Geese are viewed by most as being cold, as being not ones to show emotion. This idiosyncrasy generally makes them seem unapproachable. But the fact is that inside the snow goose is a great treasure, though it will not be had easily.

While the snow gooses grow up with the medicine of perfection, they have a difficult time fitting in with the rest of their society. When everyone is given an assignment, the snow goose is invariably the last to turn it in for evaluation. The others may rush through the project, doing just the minimum to skate by. This will puzzle the snow goose. He will be the last to turn in his work because he wants every last moment to perfect the assignment at hand.

When the snow goose's neighbor shows him their project, the snow goose will be quick to point out its flaws and weaknesses, not a quality conducive to developing friendships and relationships.

Nothing gets past a snow goose; she sees every detail. So who is good to have snow goose medicine? Accountants, organizers, people in jobs were minute details are of significant importance.

---

[25] One of the highest of all Native American ceremonies, it occurs on the Summer Solstice, around June 21st. It includes four days of dancing in the circle for our Earth Mother, and we also make a petition of our own. I have attended for many years, honoring a commitment in this way. Sundancers must give flesh and blood during this ceremony. Enough said about that.

When travelling the world to participate in many spiritual events, the two most coveted assistants prayed for are the Snow Goose and the Sturgeon. They will be my eyes and ears, to assist in Spirit's work and to give solid counsel.

At a big event, an introduction was made to a particular individual who owns thirty schools that train in metaphysics. With many distractions it could be easy to overlook this person. This is when the Snow Goose helper comes and gives a nudge and says, "See that guy in the red shirt? He has thirty metaphysical schools. You should go speak with him."

The Sturgeon helper will advise on the truth. If I am talking with a person who is making some sort of offer, the Sturgeon helper will give them the thumbs up, "Yes, he is genuine," or the thumbs down, "No, he is full of deceit and treachery."

The Sturgeon is outgoing and may appear to be demanding; however, there is much more to this fish than meets the eye.

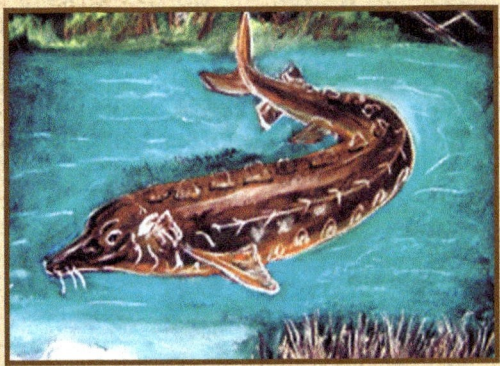

Sturgeon

Mouse

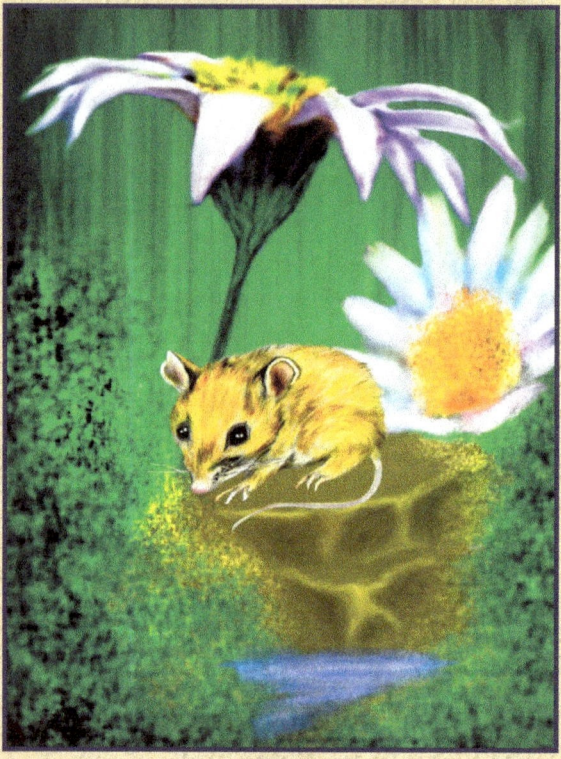

Mouse

If someone says you have mouse medicine, you may think, "Hmm… I would rather have eagle or bear medicine. It sounds more powerful."

Well, all of Creator's children have special gifts (although sometimes I wonder about mosquitoes.) Since a mouse is such a small creature, he represents the South, the place of small Four Legged people.

Take a small rock, for instance: we, as big people, would step over it with less than a thought. But a small rock is a big concern to Mr. Mouse. He has to make an important decision.

Shall he climb over the rock, or perhaps go around it, or even yet, how about digging a hole and going under it

This is 'attention to detail' medicine. Those who would benefit from such a medicine are accountants, organizers, quality technicians and inspectors.

Wolf

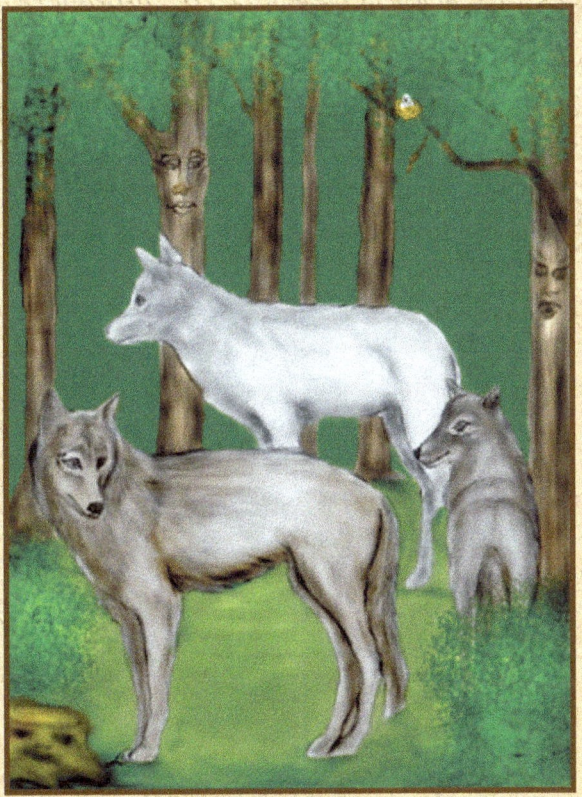

Wolves

The wolf is well known for being clever and cunning, but where does that come from? Well, if the wolf has a thing they want to do, it is not their way to just rush in and do it as the hawk would do.

Mr. Wolf and Mrs. Hawk sat down to talk. Mr. Wolf asked, "How will you accomplish this thing?" Mrs. Hawk replied, "I don't know, but I will do it, that's for sure." Mr. Wolf said, "But that doesn't make sense. You're going to do it and you don't even know how?" "Yes," replied Mrs. Hawk. "That's right."

A hawk person will decide yesterday to drive across the United States tomorrow; even though she only has enough money for gas to get halfway there, and has no spare tire, let alone a jack if there is a flat. But go the hawk does, and get there the hawk does, and all the time the wolf is scratching his head in wonder. We all have our ways.

Wolf medicine is one that says, "If I do this, than this can happen, or that can happen, or maybe that can happen, or possibly that other thing can happen." All this will then be considered prior to doing the task at hand. But that is still not good enough for the wolf. They will go over another possible avenue, and then another and another, until they are fully satisfied as to the possible outcome.

Wolverine

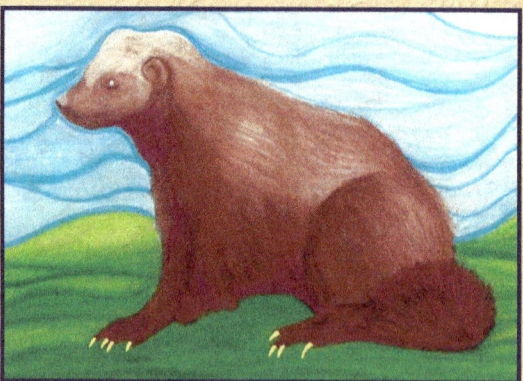

Wolverine

The power and authority of this Four Legged Person fears no one and no thing, and has final dominion over its closely guarded boundaries. The fur on the wolverine does not freeze, which indicates the medicine of survival in extreme conditions.

Fearlessness.

Turtle

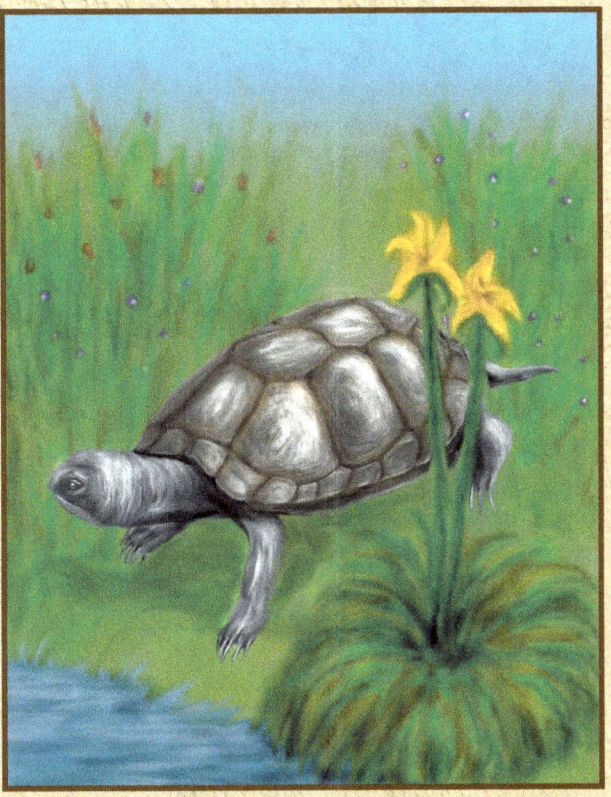

Turtle

The turtle has the medicine of tenacity and is always at home, as they carry their home upon their back. If a turtle has the mind set to walk twenty yards and half way there, she encounters a fence, it will not stop her. If the fence is twenty miles long, the turtle will walk twenty miles to where the fence begins, cross around it, walk another twenty miles back to the spot where her journey was detoured and then walk the remaining ten yards to complete her original journey.

One of the biggest hoaxes I can see on Earth these days is the calendar. Once upon a time, the Indian calendar was the turtle. Why is this and what about the future?

The shell of a desert turtle has thirteen squares on its back, each signifying the time cycle in terms of lunar months. The South Americans used this system as well as Indians, although I don't know if they used the turtle in this way or not, as my teachings are from Turtle Island[26] and not South America.

Any woman can tell you about the 28-day moon cycle which also happens inside their bodies. In thirteen cycles, the moon will return to its original position in the sky, thus completing one year. What is your truth?

Besides all of that, the turtle is a survivor. In the hot desert of the Southwest, temperatures can reach incredible highs, 130 degrees in the shade in some places. Where most other animals would perish or not even be able to exist, the turtle thrives.

The turtle is low to the ground; thus, in many tribes, the turtle represents the Earth and the medicine of the Earth.

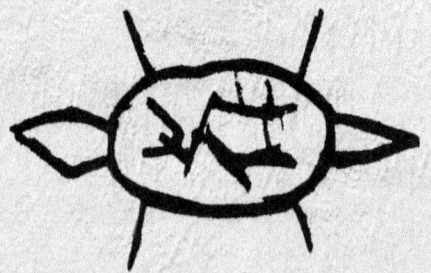

---

[26] Long ago when Indian people were sent to the four directions, they came back with geographic reports: off the East coast was Florida; off the West coast, Baja, California; off the Northwest coast, the San Juan Islands; off the Northeast coast, the North East Islands. Altogether they looked like a turtle.

Buffalo

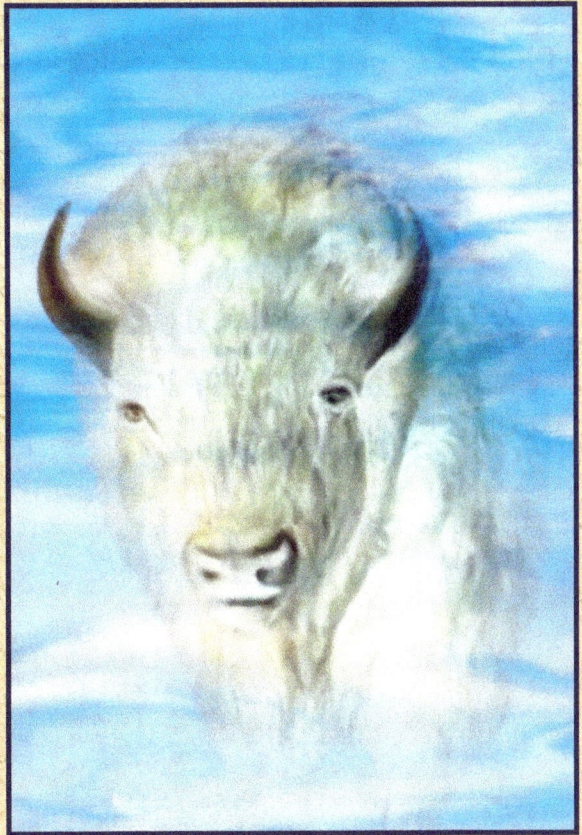

White Buffalo in the Sky

The buffalo was once the lifeline of Native American People. But people within the United States Government had some experience with colonization. They knew if they wiped out the buffalo and eliminated the Indian People's food source, then the Indian People would be dependent on the government. Perhaps the cycle will switch back some day?

On a brighter note, the "Buff" has been known as Wakan Tanka, Wakan meaning "holy" or "sacred" and Tanka meaning "buffalo." Many would associate this term, "holy buffalo", with the word "God." However, Native Americans do not consider buffalo to be God, but that's the way things go when cultures and semantics intermingle. However, the buff did supply the needs of our indigenous people once upon a time, and these days, buffaloes are making a comeback in America. Does that say something?

I heard a few years back that there was a great freeze in the Midwest. It was so cold that many of the cattle died, but the buffalo hardly diminished at all. Their meat is low in cholesterol and fat, and high in protein.

The medicine of the buffalo is that of "Spirit." The direction is North, the place of the long-haired elders and the place of wisdom (since, by this time of life, the medicine wheel has been walked upon for many seasons, bringing wisdom with it.) This is the place on the medicine wheel where we leave this world to journey to the next— the world of spirit. The buffalo has eyes that carry vision into the place of spirit, and is a sort of vehicular path to spirit and immortality.

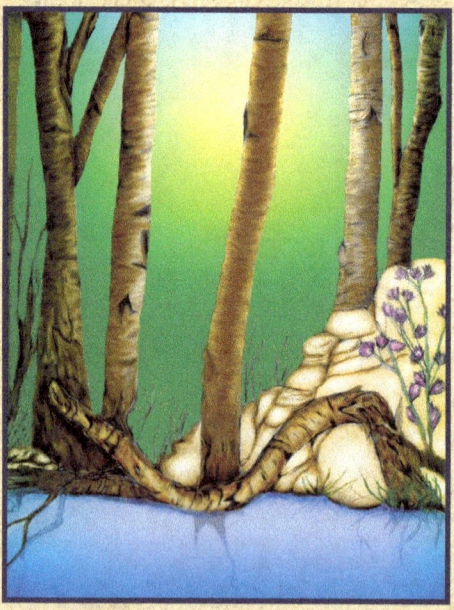

Hope

Coyote

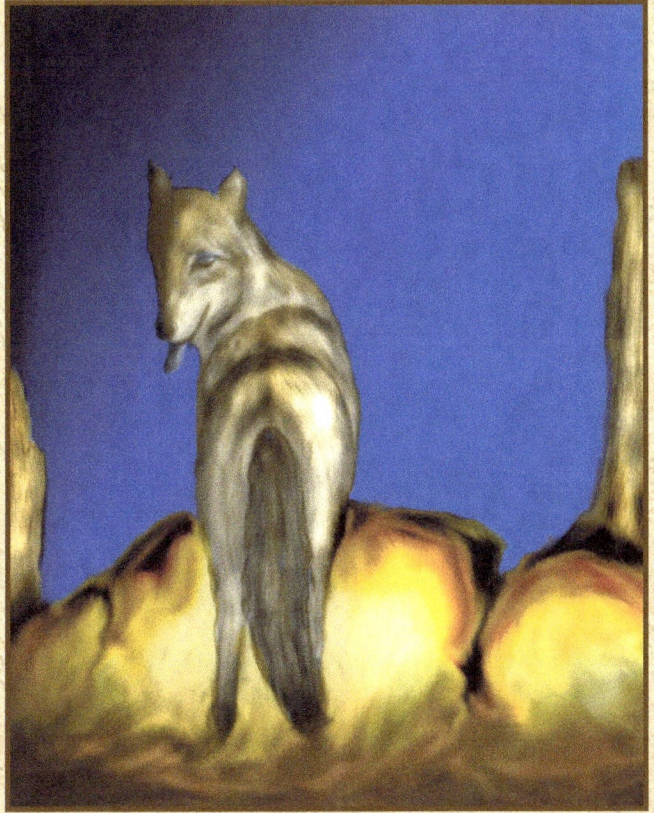

Coyote / Trickster

The coyote is the trickster; yes, most will be quick to confirm this, but the medicine of the coyote is much more than that. If there is a lesson right in front of your face and you will not see it, then that is the time the medicine of the trickster comes to guide you. So the lesson you can't or won't see is taken into the mouth of Mr. Coyote; he nips at your feet, and goes behind you swiftly and nips at your butt, purposely coaxing you into twirling around until you get dizzy. This disorientation is the opportune time for the coyote to jump you and drop the teaching/lesson right into you. Then you step back; take a breath and say, "Yes! That's the information I have been seeking and waiting for."

That is not the end of it. As the coyote has shared something of himself with you, the Indian way is to return something. In most cases, an acknowledgement of what the coyote has brought you will suffice.

This is one of the fundamental differences between western culture and indigenous cultures. Western culture is viewed as linear. A modern person receives something from Mother Earth or a medicine animal and then moves on without a thought. However, in indigenous cultures, the approach is circular. When we receive something from Mother Earth, or a gift from a totem animal or spiritual assistant, we stop and acknowledge what we have received. This completes the circle. In this way, we acknowledge All Our Relations and honour our relationships to them. Indigenous people believe that this approach of 'completing the circle' could be a benefit to many if practiced in daily life.

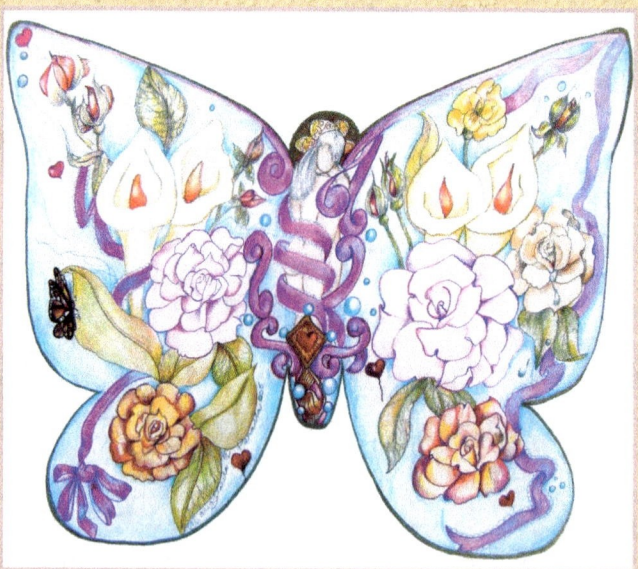

Butterfly Lovers

A young man once asked, "How do I counter coyote medicine if it is used on me?" A fair question coming from a teenager. "Use the medicine of the Water Coyote," was my response. "The Water Coyote uses water to erode the ground, the very foundation below, therefore causing the coyote to loose his footing and fall."

Rabbit

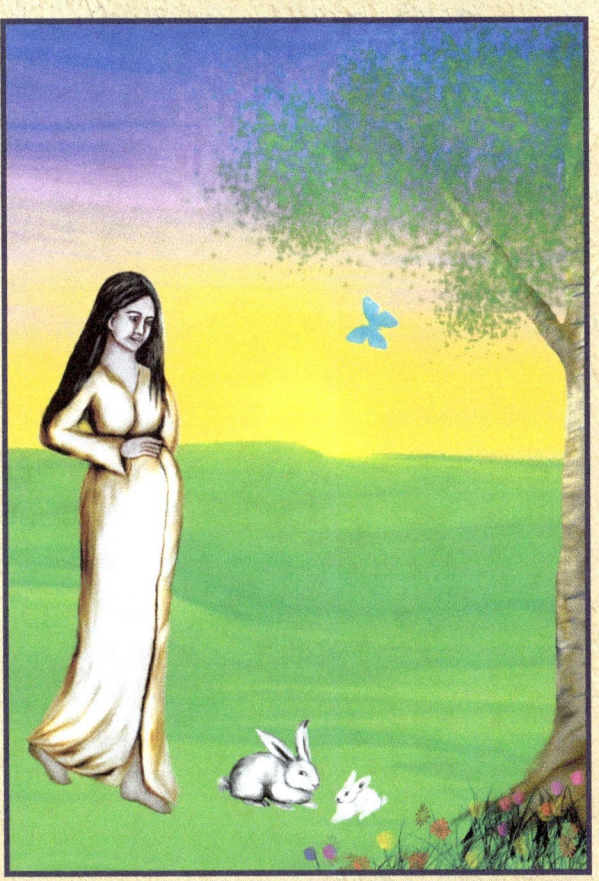

Fertility

The rabbit represents fertility, which is the key to the existence of our race. If you think of a bicycle tire, the hub holds the spokes so that the outside of the tire can have strength. The rabbit represents the hub of the wheel, the foundation that we stand upon - procreation - so that our future generations, the unborn, and what is to come, can occur. Being the foundation is the concept of the rabbit.

Eagle

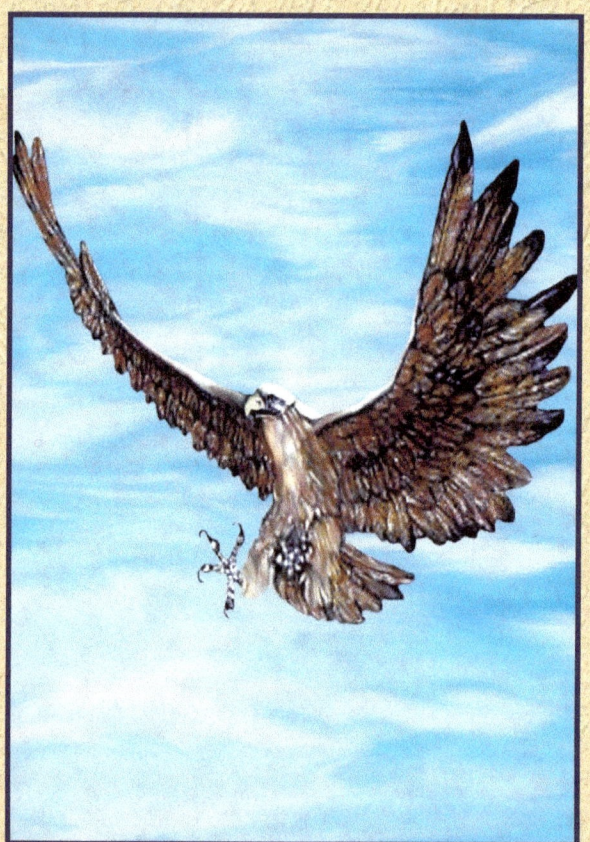

Eagle Swoops Down

This is the medicine of truth, new beginnings and the messenger. This person represents the East, the place where Grandfather Sun first shows himself. All the people of the day begin to rise here, as well. This is a time of birth, planting seeds and new orientations. Highly regarded by all Native

Americans, the eagle feather is earned by good deeds and gestures. It is given for merit and is a symbol of status. It took me a good five years to earn three eagle feathers, each gifted at a different time, while coming up through the ranks of a healer.

One time in Australia, many years into healing work, I was at my booth at a metaphysical trade show, scheduling healings for the few days following the show. A father walked by with his 16 year-old daughter. He was very loving and attentive to her and she was severely crippled; still moving on her own two legs, but with great difficulty. My heart melted and I did something I rarely do[27] I approached the man.

"Excuse me can we have a word?" I said. The father said, "Yes please." "I am a faith healer. May I be permitted to do something for your daughter?" "What do you want to do?" he asked. I replied. "If there would be one thing you would like to see in your daughter what would that be?" He thought about it and said, "She has not smiled in many years. All I ask for is one smile."

To be considerate of my fellow vendors we stepped outside. This particular situation would best be served by way of the Native American, one-sided, hand-held drum. In the close quarters of the trade show it would be too distracting or disturbing for the other vendors. I began to do a drum washing[28] on her while she stood with the father close by.

---

[27] This is the way I have been trained, and for good reason; it's not our place to be in another's personal space unless otherwise requested. But now that the books are being published, ending a more than 20-year stretch, I have hung up my healing gear in exchange for wearing the author's hat. The information gained from my experience and sacrifice are now being made available to many more people than I could reach one by one, which was the way most of these teachings were gathered.

[28] A healing technique I developed after many years of training in indigenous healing arts. It is a cleansing and balancing from within and is very powerful. I have trained and certified many of practitioners in many countries. Not an easy teaching to learn.

It took about fifteen minutes but it worked. When the drum washing was finished, she smiled, just as her father had asked. The man was beside himself, tears rolling down his cheeks. He looked at me with grateful eyes and said, "For this I will give you 100 eagle feathers." With a nod of the head in acknowledgement, it was shortly dismissed as nonsense.

When the metaphysical conference was over and packing up was almost done, the father showed up with a long thin box. When he opened it, there were 111 eagle feathers[29] and a host of other exotic bird feathers inside. I asked no questions, remembering what my father had often told me growing up, "Son don't look a gift horse in the mouth. Just say thank you."

Spider

Grandmother Spider, as our ancient oral tradition has preserved in time, says she emerged from spider rock in the Grand Canyon[30].

From her teachings come many of the things we take for granted on a daily basis. Weaving was learned by studying how she makes her web. From her matriarchal stance came the knowledge of cohesive life, of making clothes and shelters, dream catchers and buildings, seat covers, how to climb, and so much more.

She is highly respected. When one of my teachers does his spring-cleaning, he vacuums all the old spider webs out of his house careful not to harm even a baby, so that they will build a new spider web for the new season. We are talking serious infestation here, but when I stayed there, they never

---

[29] Most of these feathers were used in Byron Bay, Australia for a prayer tree at a ceremony called "Gan-da-lee," meaning "heat waves of the sun." It is also called "the horse dance" because it is done in the shape of a horseshoe with four choices or paths representing the four directions, kind of like a rainbow.
[30] A place truly worthy of a visit. It is located in Arizona and is easily accessible by car.

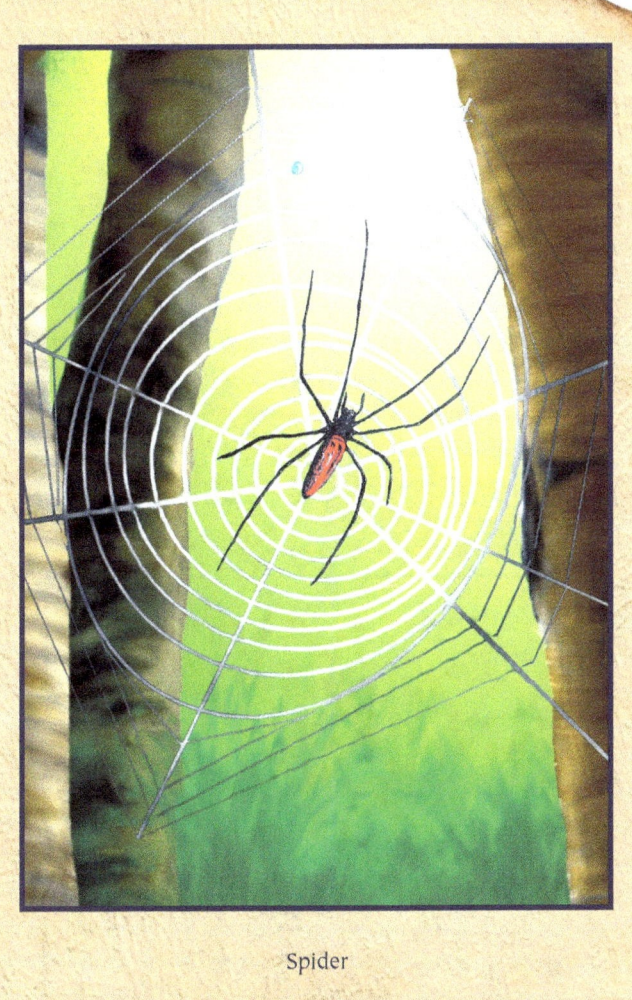

Spider

bothered me and we eventually became friends. Some very interesting insects are referred to as "Many Legged People."

Have a go at it sometime. Sit still, not disturbing them, and take a long look. View with your Universal Vision, listen with your Universal Hearing and open your senses to all, from the light that serves the higher good.

Animal Medicine and You

These are Native American teachings, but you have the power to elicit animal medicines, I promise you. If you are not familiar with that which extends beyond these few animals, that is OK because your medicine is far stronger than mine. If you chose to say so . . .

So you may watch whatever animals you choose, digest what they have taught you and look within yourself to find your own answers. As long as you ask in a good way and with a good heart, all will be fine, and you, too, can pull upon your bloodlines and diverse heritages facilitated by these teachings. Dare to!

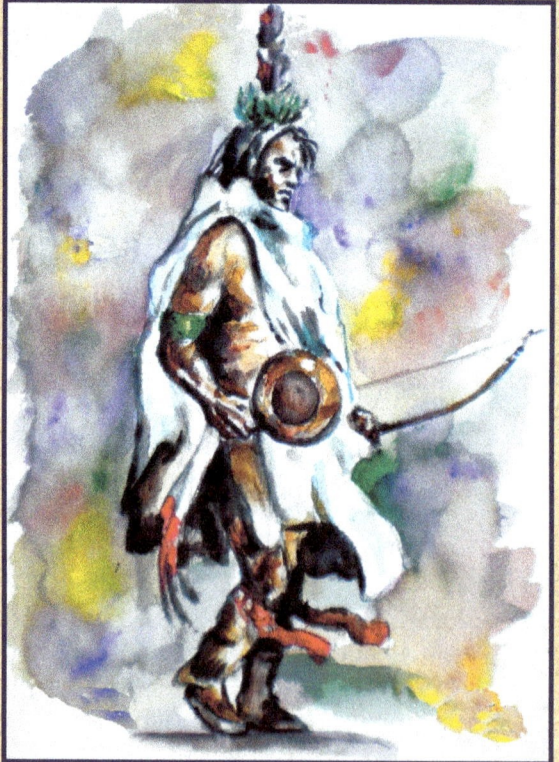

Ceremonial Dancer

SPIRIT GUIDES

Spirit guides can be quite misunderstood outside of indigenous cultures because of a fear of the unknown. Some people may assume that things beyond their vision are dark in nature. Here is an attempt to clear up the lack of knowledge in this area.

Spirit guides are synonymous with angels and everyone is assigned one at birth. People usually ask me, "Is it a person? Is it a blood relative? Do they have wings? Do they live in the spirit world or what?"

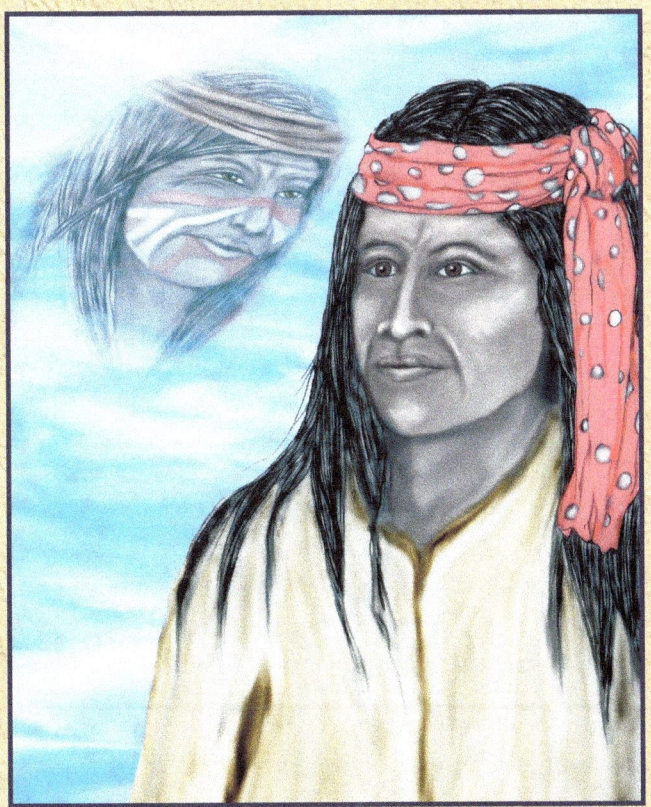

Whispers

The way it works is that one spirit guide has you as an assignment. Their job is to guide you on your path according to the contract you made before you came here and were birthed by your mother.

Spirit guides walk with you for your entire life and it's your choice whether you listen to them or not. It really is the listener's choice. They are talking anyway, but whether you listen or not, well, that's up to you.

Spirit guides have something like helicopter vision; they can see things that are coming up on your horizon. Knowing your future, they provide tools for you. What is going to happen is inevitable, whether you want it to happen or not. So it is their job to make sure you do what you are supposed to do. This means future tools.

Whether you accept the tool or not is up to you. If you accept it, then when the event happens you will have the tool your spirit guide believes will behoove you to have in order for you to grow from that experience.

Some people have said, "You say I only have one spirit guide but I'm sure I have three." It is possible to have three spirit guides. The situation is that your one spirit guide called in the other two, depending on the nature of the project.

Then they say, "But the three of them have been with me for ten years." And I say, "Fine, then your project ain't done yet, pardon my French." You may have three spirit guides until the particular mission is accomplished, then the other two will go away, leaving the one who will always be with you

Your spirit guide will guide you on the path determined by the season of the year you were born in. There are four seasons, each corresponding to one of the four directions, and each season is split into three parts. When you get your spirit guide, they know the one medicine you received from your birth direction. Then they assist you in gaining the medicine from the other three directions; that is one of their missions. The path to enlightenment is in discovery of all four directions.

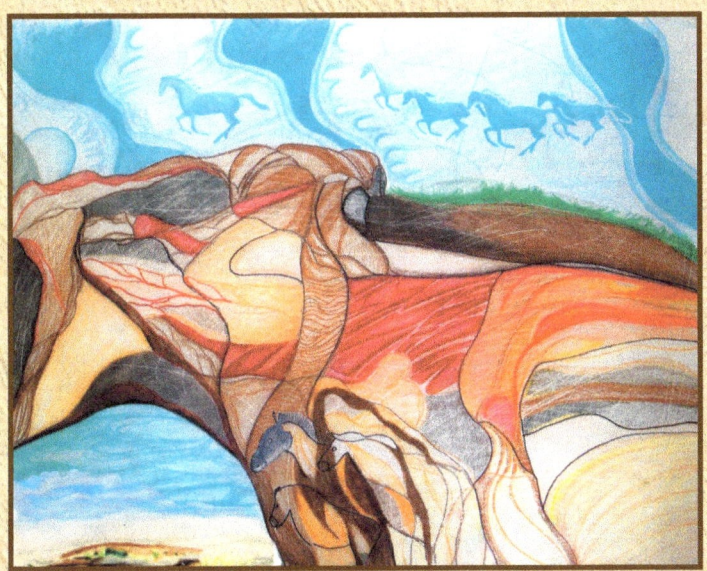

Horses

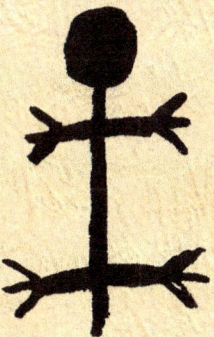

COLORS AND THEIR MEDICINES

According to Native American beliefs, colors have power and authority, and attributes with specific representations. Knowing this material can shed light on alternative ways to evoke light spirits. This is the best generalization of accepted teachings that I am capable of at this time, so enjoy it and keep an open mind, as your benefit may then be optimal. There will be diverse teachings according to the different regions of Turtle Island, but the teachings are conceptual and your medicine is stronger than my medicine.

The main idea is the four directions are represented by colors. Most tribes subscribe to four directions; some subscribe to five and some even subscribe to seven.

Yellow

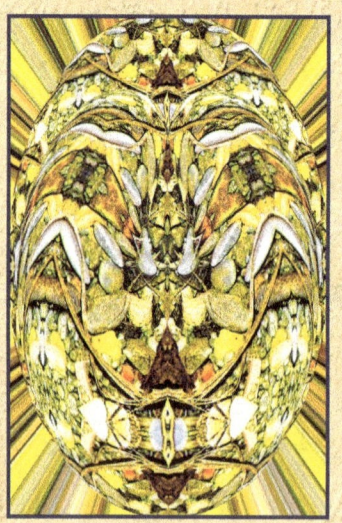

Yellow

Yellow represents the direction of the East and the people of the East (the Yellow People.) As understood from my teachers and my years of experience as a Spiritual Advisor of the Red Road[31], at the time that Creator put the four races on Earth Mother, he also designated their attributes.

The shade of yellow generally accepted in this regard looks

---

[31] Red Road is a common term that refers to the red man, red skin, red blood, red heart and red Earth, signifying the Indian way of life, the harmony of living in sync with "All My Relations." In fun, some say "it's the Pow Wow Highway", for those who follow the Pow Wow circuit which is basically seasonal.

like gold, such as the golden sunrise that happens so often on Turtle Island.

As the color yellow is associated with the East, the place of new beginnings, truth, birth, and the planting of seeds, so, yellow is also linked to hope; we see the first sign of the new day in the sunlight shining through the mist of the dark forest, before the sun comes up.

Red

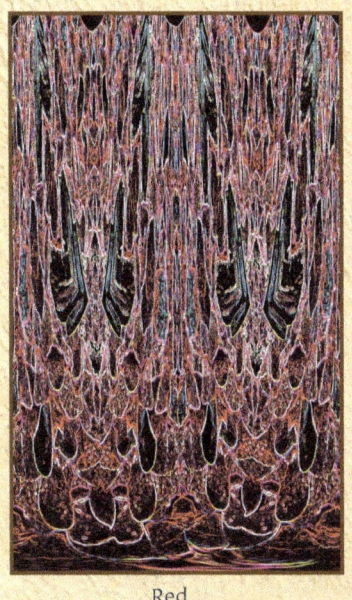

Red

Moving in a clockwise fashion, the next direction is South and the color is red. This color represents bottlenose dolphins as well as small four-legged animals such as the mouse, turtle, and squirrel.

As the South is the place of youth and vitality, red also represents raging hormones and impatience, since youth always seem to need things to be "in the now." Some may feel bravery at this age; most would feel their- selves to be invincible, immune from the effects of non-pubescent adults. This strength can be called upon, be specific.

Red is the color of our blood, us, the Two Legged ones. This represents the connectedness of many relatives and can show the trail to world peace if you are willing to see it.

Red is the color of the pipestone we use to make the bowls of our most sacred Chinupa[32] (peace pipe.) It has been said that the pipestone only lives in one place in the world, Pipestone, Minnesota. I have been there and it is full of distinct energies. If you have one, it is only for your private use.

The South is a place to ask the Grandmothers and Grandfathers for assistance in ways that are concerned with the medicine of the South, as is true when asking for assistance with matters pertaining to any particular direction.

Black

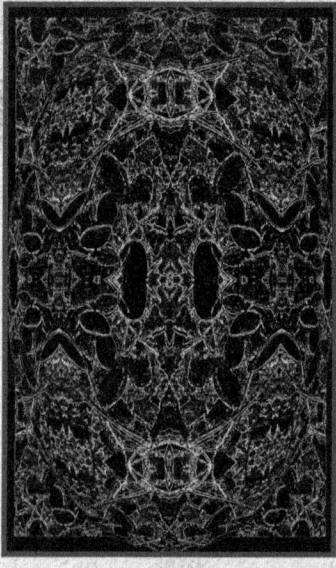

Black

The next color is black. Black represents purification and healing,[33] as well as the fruits that come in great seasonal quantities. It also represents Young Elders; they do not quite have all the wisdom yet, but enough to show some white hair to all.

The animals that correspond to this color are the vulture, the one who cleans up Mother Earth; and the bear, who signifies the "looks with-in" medicine of introspection.

The direction is the West, the place where rest begins as Grandfather Sun sets and leaves us with the blackness of night. This is also the place where Grandmother Moon comes to share her medicine with all. Life begins to slow down. We now take the time to smell the flowers once again. The

---

[32] The pipe is carried by those who have undergone Spiritual practice sufficient enough to deem them worthy of such an honor.
[33] Although this color represents healing and purification, I strongly recommend that black feathers not be used in healings, protection, or purification!

willingness to graciously accept the rewards that now come as a result of being a good "keeper" of all.

White

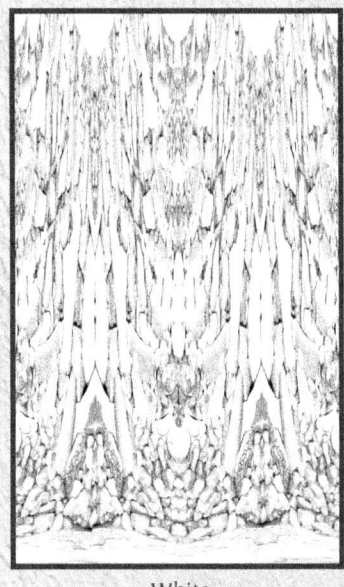

White is the color of wisdom and spirit. It corresponds to the direction of the North, where things tend to be white for long periods of time. It is the place of rest and rejuvenation.

White is the collection of all colors, so it represents wholeness and gratitude.

The color white is also represented by quartz, whose medicine is the retention of memory, kind of like the whales are our record keepers. It is also representative of spotted dolphins, the spiritual leaders of the oceans. The buffalo is dominant in the North, which is depicted as white; both signify Spirit. When the blanket of snow keeps all below in a state of rest and replenishing that is the time of the North. When it is our time to journey to the next world we leave from the North. There are a few things that can be taken on that journey and one of them is your spiritual bank account.

White

Blue

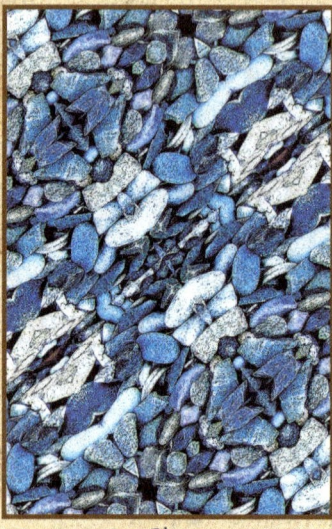

Blue

For tribes who subscribe to seven directions, the fifth direction is represented by the color blue. This is the direction of above, of the sky, and all that entails.

All that is applicable to Creator is also held within the attributes/medicine of this direction: Spirit, divinity, Shangri La, Heaven, Nirvana, etc. This concept is uniquely illustrated in the Wisdom Cards[34].

For those tribes subscribing to five directions, green is the color that corresponds to the fifth direction. However, and this is somewhat of a complicated concept, blue is also in there in relationship to green. In calling in the fifth direction upon Mother Earth, the connection could extend below into green infinity and above into blue infinity. Thus, green is the color of the fifth direction, and blue comes into play in relation to it.

[34] *I do not necessarily condone tarot cards and the like, so one day I was given an assignment to do something about it. Based on teachings, I was blessed to lead and participate in medicine ways, which resulted in a series of 52 cards. The artistic renditions are used for divination of the future and were specifically developed to assist snake people (basically Scorpios) in their work as healers. The goal was to provide a beautiful artistic rendition of Native American based Wisdom and Teachings. Available on the web site www.2feather.com.*

Purple

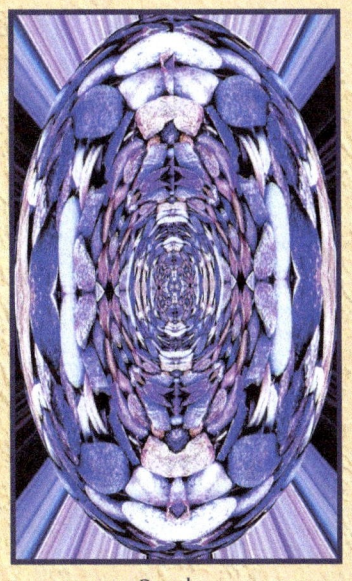

Purple

Purple is only used in the seven color applications. It is the place where Spirit lives, represented by the dragonfly and the hummingbird. These small ones are suspended between Mother Earth and the sky, where Creator lives. Their little hearts beat very fast and they are delicate and gentle[35].

It is interesting to note that "blue ray youth," also called "crystal kids" and 'Indigo Children"[36] respond to the color purple, or indigo. So if you feel the need to connect to spirit, wearing purple or having something purple in your general area is a good way to do this. It works according to the vibrational frequency emitted by the color, so even if you wear something purple underneath your visible clothing, it will still increase spiritual matters by its presence, and still be a draw.

Amethyst is the stone appropriate to this area of discipline. If people dislike this color, it sometimes raises the question why, like the smoke of sage. The home of Spirit is as large as the world we live in everyday. There is a hierarchy. There are jobs that need to be done and things that need to be tended to on a regular basis. As it is above, so it is below.

---

[35] In no way does this mean that spirit must be delicate or gentle. It does not make logical sense, so take it for what it's worth. Go figure.
[36] One way to identify Indigo children is to have my assistant dress in all purple, which attracts the indigo youth. They will usually come right up, hug the assistant, and thus identify themselves. Look up Drumvalo Melchizedek, Kryon, or Gregg Braden for more information.

Green

For tribes who subscribe to five directions, the fifth direction is represented by the color green. For tribes subscribing to seven directions, the color green represents the seventh direction.

Green signifies both the Earth, our Mother, and all who live below, as well as the sky. Yes, most tribes believe that there are people who live in the Earth. Some believe in one race and some believe there are many races.

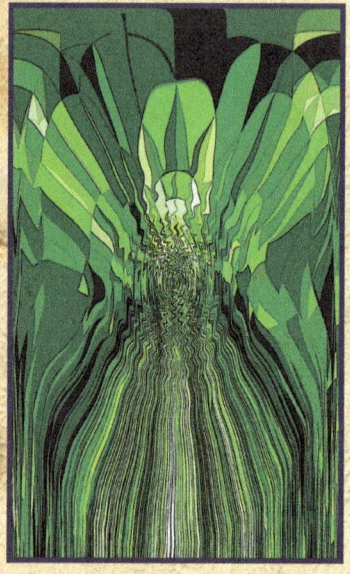

Green

Green is also the color of 'twin flame' people, those who have two medicines ~ male physical attributes and a female

personality, or vice versa. These people were not feared within Indian communities in times of old. They served vital roles, one of which was to stay behind when the Braves went to raid, hunt, or fight in battles to count coup.[37] The twin-flame men stayed behind to guard the women, children and old men. While the Braves where away tending to their duties, they had no concerns about the fidelity of their women with twin-flame men on guard.

When calling in protection, I tend to use the color green, with all its power and authority to represent all that our Mother Earth does; I fill my protection circle with this cool hue (using visualization.) Can you visualize ice cream on a sunny day?

---

[37] *This is a term used in battle - see reference in glossary.*

SACRED NUMBERS

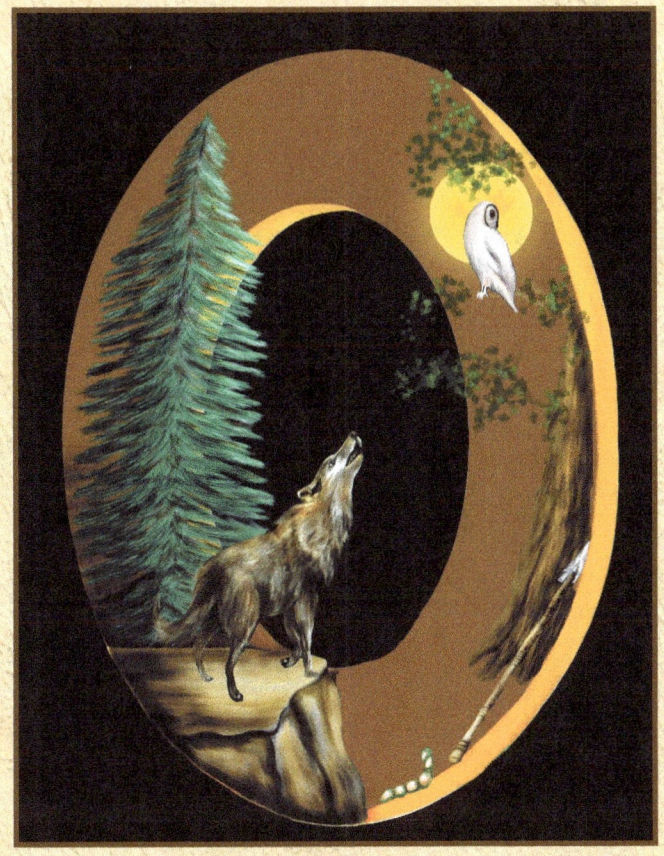

"O"

Native American lore is not well known for mathematics; nevertheless, it is part of our life and, in fact, a system was and is still in use in many places. I like to refer to this as 'Native American Sacred Geometry,' (N.A.S.G.)

To begin with, numbers have different prescribed values than those commonly assigned to it in western terms.

ZERO is the essence of our way of life. It is the Medicine Wheel of life. It denotes that all things have substance; the circle has no beginning and no end and, in a loose interpretation, so does life. Although we did have a beginning and that was when Creator made us Two Leggeds into four races and put us in the four directions. Numerically speaking, the circle always IS, and so, too, is life.

The next sacred number is ONE. That means us; we are one with everything. Knowledge of this has the potential to foster the positive aspect in our societies of mutual respect[38], or, at least, tolerance. We say it as "All My Relations," one more thing that we as a Red Race of People can contribute to the world. We are one with everything and, in so being, we show the value of respect, a strong foundation for world peace, tolerance, and what is right.

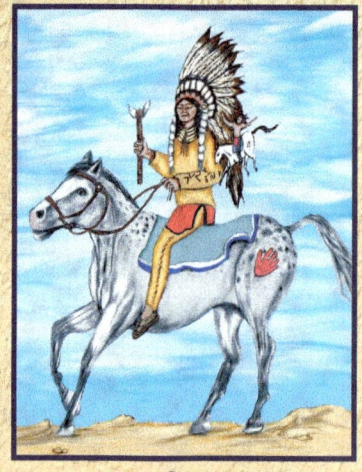

One

As a sacred number, TWO is noteworthy for delineating marriage, the sacred bond between two people, referred to as "half sides." In order to be half sides, two people form a sacred bond of oneness, proclaimed for all to witness during the sacred bonding ceremony.[39] Once the bond has been made, the two can still maintain their autonomy. They are two individuals with two identities that have made the choice to become one.

---

[38] *The Japanese Indians, who were forced to live in the inhospitable North, have a matriarchal society. Grandmother Be Good is the Matriarch and has had a ceremony every year for many years. At night, they do not go out around sundown as not to disturb the animals during dinner time. They are called Ainu, pronounced, "I-knew." Grandmother's other name is Ashiri Rera.*
[39] *I have been performing marriage rites for many years and in many countries. The two kiss under a blanket after drinking from a sacred vessel with two sides. This signifies that from now on, these two will partake from the same cup of life.*

There is a duality within us of good and bad. At any moment, the balance can shift to either side; the side we feed naturally becomes the strongest. It's your choice who you will feed.

One of the cards in the Wisdom Deck (for divination of the future) is a warrior riding on a fine pony with a Mini-Me suspended in mid-air at his left shoulder. The Mini-Me is reaching into the back of the Brave's head. This card represents the duality within. The card itself has been given the numerical spoken value of one; however the depiction of the warrior and his mini-me also illustrates a deeper meaning of the number two. From one, two will come; aka mitosis?

THREE is sacred as it delineates the Two Leggeds. It has long been recognized that Native Americans refer to a person as being made up of integral parts mind, body, and spirit. In Western terms, a human is a body only. What effect might it have to share the Native American's teachings of the three aspects of self in today's educational system? That is food for thought. You may notice that braids are made of three parts woven together as one.

FOUR is sacred as it speaks of the four directions, each of which has Grandmothers and Grandfathers who tend to it and share its knowledge. Derivatives of four[40] carry the same weight as represented by the four sacred directions. Some people say with condemning voices, "Oh, you Indians have a ceremony for everything." Well, we don't actually, but we do have a lot of ceremony in our lives. It seems to be one of the main bonding components lacking in modern society. When a boy reaches manhood, what acknowledgements do modern societies have for this very special time of transition? Hmm. Most Tribes have some

---

[40] Derivatives of four are generally in the low multiples of four.

form of ceremonial acknowledgement, though in varying time frames, methodologies and ideologies.

In a world were many indigenous societies are dwindling and many are even facing extinction, procreation is critically important to the very survival of the race. Native Americans believe that Creator tells us it is time for a woman to get ready to be married soon after she has had her first moon time. [41]If a woman goes many years without a husband after her moon time has begun, this is a not such a good thing. The father and mother wish grandsons and granddaughters to carry on the bloodline to ensure a foundation for the future.

When we plant seeds, we expect them to grow and yield fruit sometime in the future. If the seeds are not planted properly, the fruits may not have the opportunity to grow. Therefore, if youth do not know when they have moved from one phase of life to another phase of life, from boy to man, from girl to woman, that can leave them with a very insecure foundation. An insecure foundation leads to an insecure future.

It is an important responsibility of ours, as teachers, grown-ups, and guides, that we point our young people in the direction that will best serve them. This will allow them to have a better foundation to stand upon in order to serve themselves and all people in the future. So it is in everyone's best interest to see to it that our youth have the strongest foundations possible, because someday, when we are the ones with long white hair, these former youth will then be the ones calling the shots about our destiny.

As it stands today, the seeds we are planting are money

---

[41] *Moon time is the common reference in Native culture for menstruation; the time of youth no more, and the onset of womanhood and Creator's blessing to give life.*

and greed, such as putting growth hormones into our cows to yield more meat in order to make more money. But the other side of this coin shows us that when we put growth hormones into fast food products like hamburgers and hot dogs, young people eat these products and get the growth hormones inside them. Then they start developing at a faster rate than Creator says they should rightfully be growing at. When they are hurried up early in life, they don't have a chance later in life to develop according to the natural order of the universe. So here we see a glimpse of the fruit that may be yielded in the future according to the seeds we are planting today. This we call "Hawks-Vision."

Indian people suggest to all peoples of the world that before you take an action, consider first the consequences it will have for three generations to come.

FIVE is sacred in that to some tribes it delineates the directions. The four directions we are most familiar with are East, West, South and North. The fifth direction is Earth Mother and all who live above and below. In societies who subscribe to the five directions, this doctrine is usually leaned upon heavily in life and in regard to ceremony.

SEVEN is sacred in that it delineates the seven directions. Some four directional tribes use seven directions for spiritual connotations from time to time.

EIGHT has great significance, as it is two zeros, one on top of the other, and is a close derivative of four.

TWELVE is the number of change. Wherever or whenever you are in a group with this number of people, my teachers remind me to "pay attention" because a change is at hand.

As far as I have been taught, that is basically the extent of the order of sacred numbers, for these basic teachings.

Native Americans also use numbers to delineate life according to the number of legs we have: one, two, four, or many. The insects are referred to as many leggeds, and are also fondly referred to as "creepy crawlers." When legs do not apply, then another physical characteristic may be used, or maybe the place where one lives, such as "the winged people" (birds), or "the people who live in the ocean and breathe air" (mammals), and the rest of the "water people" (ocean.)

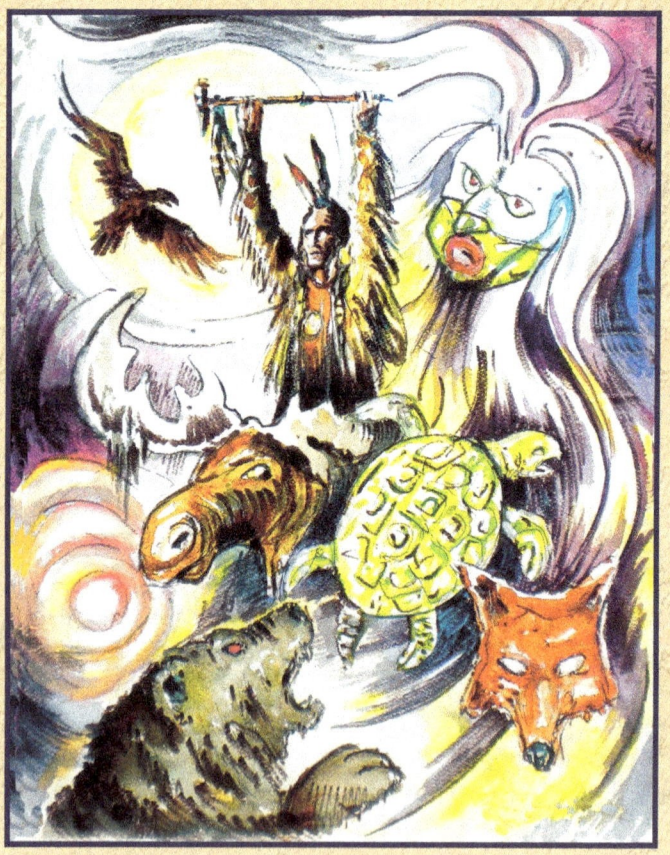

Shaman of The North

CONCEPTUAL PRAYERS
ARE POWERFUL

In the conceptual arena of prayer, we would pray for the feeling of the arm reaching for a cool drink on a hot summer day in the middle of the desert. That feeling represents the conceptual aspect of praying for what you need, or what you believe you want.

Pray for the feeling of that arm as it extends out to a brother or sister in a gesture of friendship and kindness.

This is a time when you might be asking, "What if I do it wrong? I don't know how to do such things." Know that it is already within you. Trust in yourself; stand in your own power.

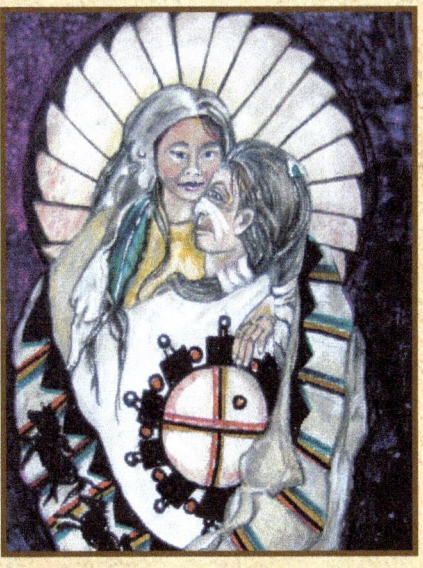

The Embrace

Acknowledge that you are not just a pawn, not a mere instrument or just a channel. You are an integral part of the process, not to be demeaned or left out of the accolades. In this sense, one individual is not everything but an important fragment of everything.

Keeping the ego within tolerable levels is part of the checks and balance system, to assist us to stay in line, flying straight. Your Own Medicine is stronger than mine and your medicine is as strong as that of Jesus Christ; He said that himself, as have other great teachers.

UNIVERSAL TRUTHS

Great teachers have similar beliefs. Some traditional stories of the Yellow People tell of such teachings from their "Wise Ones." Many other societies have similar beliefs, too. I refer to this as a "Universal Truth."

This concept can easily be realized by considering a short notion; see yourself sitting by a still pond. It is early morning and the water appears as smooth as glass.

There is a rock protruding from the edge of the pond, out over the water. You stand upon the rock and with your hand, you tap the water gently. As a result, ripples go out in precise circles. The circles are what are obvious; and the circle is the principle foundation of the Native American Way. Consider how many ripples go out from one tap on the water, and you can gain insight into the universe.

Consider beyond this, and as the ripples flow outward, draw a line that silhouettes their fluid movement and it looks like a radio wave. If you haven't seen a radio wave, think of the rolling waves of the ocean. They form a similar pattern that also looks like a flowing motion. No matter what country you are in, or what language you speak, this motion will be the same. Thus, this is one of the Universal Truths. Granted, they are few and far between, but some do exist.

The power of prayer has no limits. You might say your imagination is the only limit, but even that limit cannot come close to holding back in any significant way the awesome potential of your true power.

Students coming into their power do not have to go too fast. They should take a breath before taking too big of a leap, pause, and pray hard for the strength to do what needs to be done. There is plenty enough time, and so "all things in their own time."

Different Countries

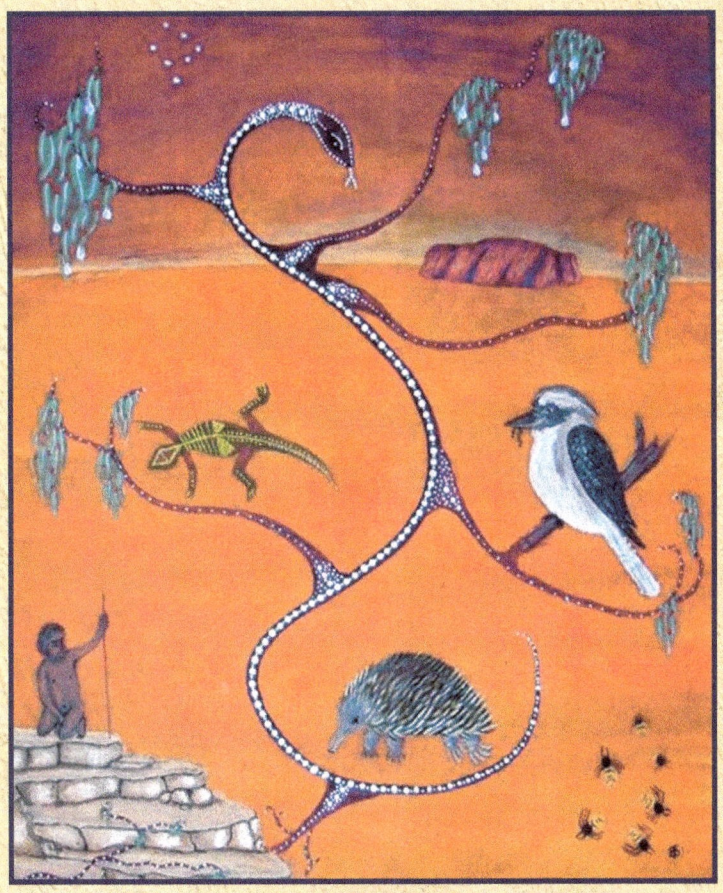

Walk About

What happens when these Native American medicinal applications are practiced in other countries? We all have to concede that water drains clockwise in the northern hemispheres, and in the southern hemisphere, water drains counter-clockwise, as was discovered on my first trip to Australia.

This question was not one that could be asked of my teachers since none of them had ever left the United States to practice traditional faith healing (medicine) in other countries.

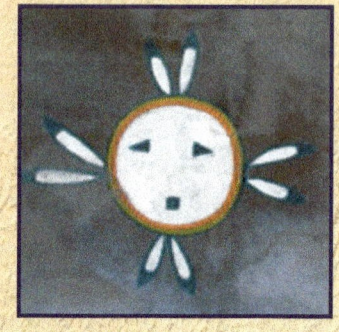

Petroglyph Face

So in this light, how does the medicine of animals work? It was a concern of mine as I approached the southern hemisphere for the first time, intentioned on doing healing work on their people.

Carrying medicine tools from country to country is a problem in itself, but I had no idea what lay in store for me at the airport going through Australian customs! That's a story in itself; but suffice it to say that every single immigration person even remotely linked to the department that day was present at my inquisition, it was three hours before I got out of the airport, and the airport was empty by then. Nothing was disturbed and all were respectful, except for the initial officer, who was new to the job. All the medicine tools passed inspection, though the most difficult one to deal with was a bit of soil in a medicine bag around my neck. The special dirt in that medicine pouch had come from Chimayo, a Holy Place and one of very few in the world recognized by the Catholic Church as a place of Miracles. I ate the dirt and that solved the problem.[42]

---

[42] *Chimayo is near my home in northern New Mexico. I am referring to geophagia: the practice of eating dirt from a sacred area to receive miraculous results. There is a room in a church at Chimayo with numerous wheelchairs, crutches and stretchers, all left behind by believers who walked out on their own two feet, miraculously cured. Two ley lines of electromagnetic energy intersect there causing the area to vibrate at a particular frequency, as, for instance, the vibration of the musical note F or F sharp specifically helps to heal the heart. This place in Chimayo alters the chemical composition of the body: the estrogen, testosterone, serotonin, etc.*

So the mystery was solved ~ upon practicing Indigenous Native American Healing techniques from the Northern hemisphere, they worked just fine. Here is a good place to note that Spirit knows neither time nor space; that is generally accepted amongst Spiritual Disciplines as a fundamental fact.

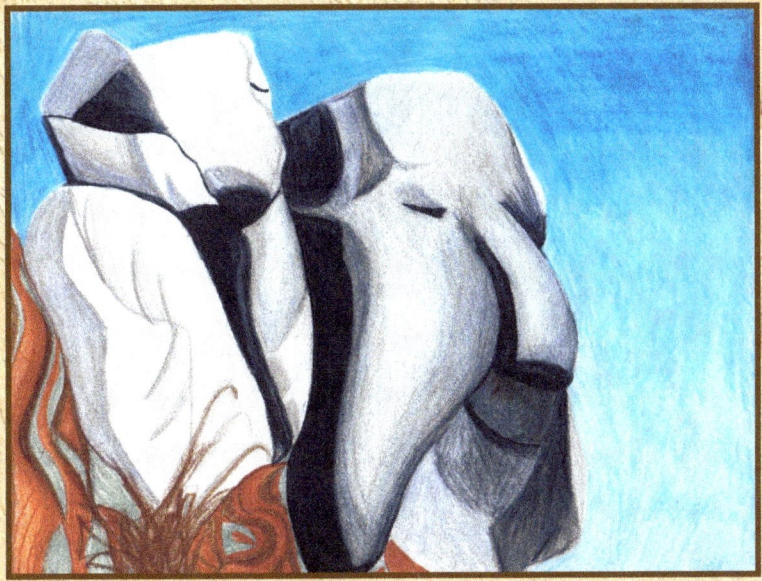
Ancestors

The concern was since some things below the equator have different flows or energies. So use "heyoka" or not? Turns out the medicine worked the same, so all is well.

HEALER, HEAL THYSELF ~ THEN HEAL OTHERS

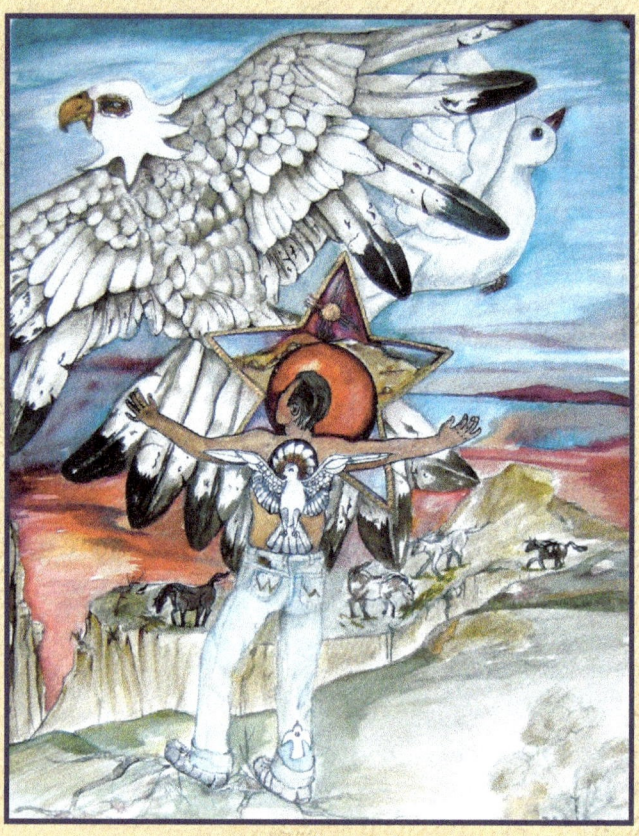

Man + Good = Eagleman

I can remember an incident with one of my three teachers. He had become ill and lost a lot of weight. He had to take some injections of "white brother" medicine every day. After a few years of this, his skin had changed color and his clothes were falling off due to weight loss. It appeared to me that the time could be drawing near for him to journey to the next world. There was a burning question that needed to be asked, but it was of a very delicate nature. I attempted to get the question out, only making partial sentences while scrambling for the right way to be respectful. Finally he said, "You got something on your chest, well get it off and just say it like it is!'

"If you say so," I replied, referring to him as I do, "Hittalli, you don't look so good these days and you're not getting any younger." And I went on…

His face began to get red and his attitude escalated by leaps and bounds till he just exploded at me, stomping his feet and slamming his fist on the table and kicking chairs. "So you're putting me in the grave before my time so you can have my medicine, are you?"

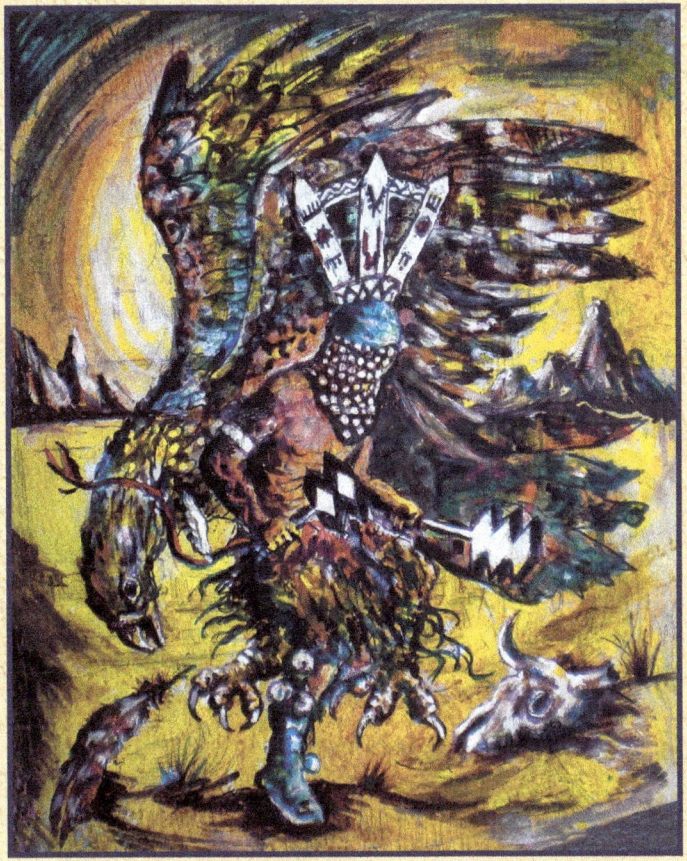

Ghan Dancer

This response was somewhat expected. And saying, "I have been with you for many years and feel that this has been earned."

He calmed down eventually, though it did not come easily or in short order. He said, "Sit down, my son; we need to talk about this!"

We sat. He said, "My medicine is strong for sure, and you have seen me cure things that the white doctors say are impossible to cure."

"Yes," I replied.

"My medicine serves me. And, yes, I can pass it on to you, but it can only serve you in a limited way, since it is mine. My place is to show you your own medicine and to bring you into your own power. That is why we (your teachers) are here; your medicine is much stronger than my medicine."

Once again I made a bad move and said, "This cannot be. I have seen what you have done for others."

He jumped up and said, "I am the teacher here. I say what, when and how much, you don't tell me." Its times like these to just be humble, obedient, shut up, and say no more.

I sure got the song and dance routine so I shut up and said no more.

After months of deep meditation on what my teacher had told me, I came to realize that my medicine was stronger than his medicine, and that the way for me to develop it was to come into my own power, not to receive from another.

It was a great day of lessons; not an easy one, but a meaningful one, as were many of the other days we shared together over the years.

THE MECHANICS OF PRAYER
A Spiritual Epiphany

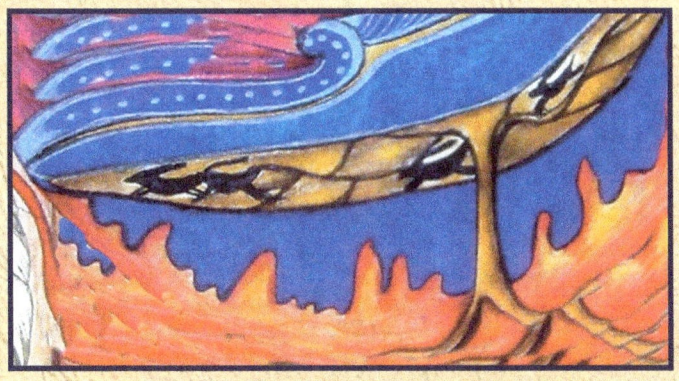

Surreal Landscape

One time, while in a deep state of spiritual connection a year or two into professional healing work, a question was asked of spirit. Spirit answered metaphorically, "I cannot pick the ball up and throw it at the target. You must do that and I, spirit, can then direct it to the center."

As Creator has made all things, each has its own particular medicine. For example, in the rock peoples' world, quartz crystal retains memory (just as memory inside a computer is stored in quartz.)

To translate this concept of medicine into plant people, let's look at tobacco. Like quartz, tobacco retains memory. So when tobacco is used in praying, the prayer is intentioned into the tobacco. How does one do this? Well, one way is to use two of the most powerful tools a person has, Will & Manifestation.

Sometimes things can be so simple. In using prayer in healing work, there is a type of mechanics, a literal ABC kind of process. Think about knowledge as having power; there are actual steps for you the seeker, dig deep, stop and think to your core. See inside.

Step 1: Setting An Intention

One of the first things to do is to get yourself squared away as a person of prayer before you jump into the work you need to do. I find that if you set an intention and purify yourself, you will be incorporating Will and Manifestation, two tools that can be merged into prayer to help you accomplish the prime directive, the main mission, which is to do the best job you can possibly do in service to others.

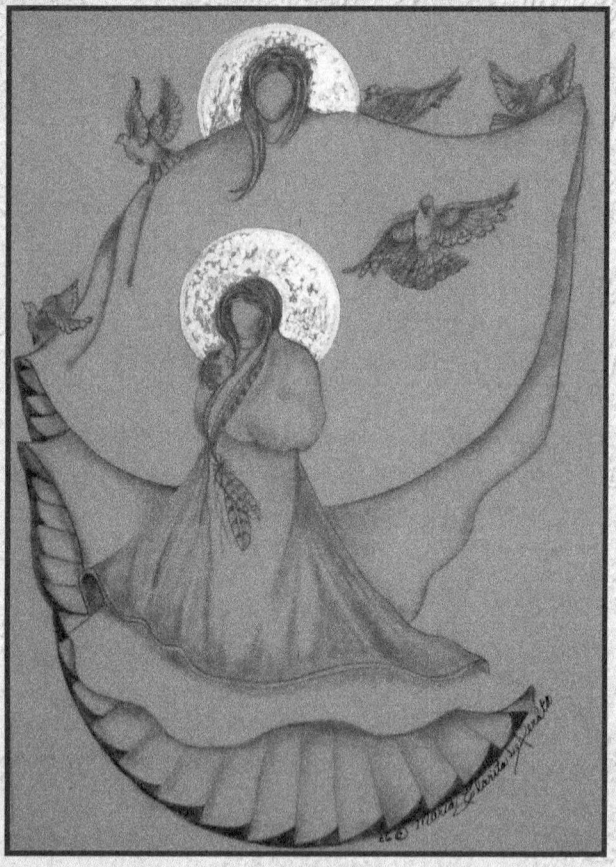

Visited by Angels

This approach to healing work can be applied to all facets of life: do the best job you can possibly do. This refers to the way you deal with a client who has come to be healed (or fixed, depending on semantics) as well as the way you deal with yourself. The more you put into your prayer projects and your life projects, the more the outcomes will reflect your desired conclusions just like planting a seed.

With this approach in mind, set an intention for this time of prayer. The intention of "the highest good of all" is recommended.

Step 2: Calling in Plant Medicine

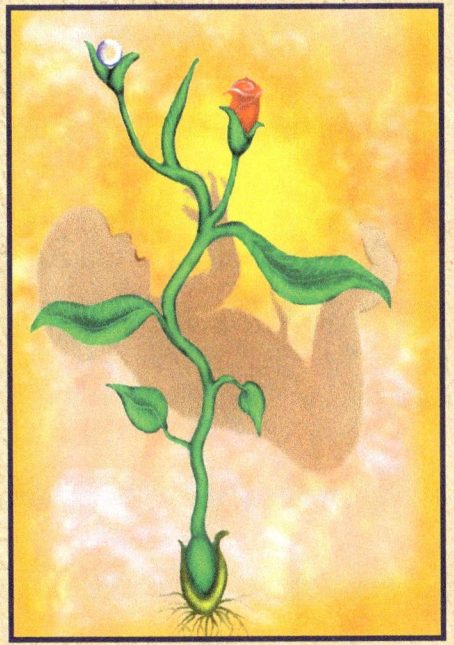

Seedling

Next, it is a good idea to call in the power and authority of the plant people, such as sage or cedar, to provide purification and protection. To do this, light the sage or cedar (beware cedar smoke is toxic so do not breathe it in.) Pass the smoke around your whole body (within twelve inches or so), paying particular attention to the bottoms of your feet. Sage is anti-bacterial and a disinfectant. It kills germs in all three realms therefore attending to all needs.

As Two Leggeds on this Earth, we are made of three aspects: Mind, Body and Spirit. We, the people of faith, subscribe to this concept. Using will and manifestation, say, "I will myself to be purified, therefore I am!"

Step 3: Acknowledging the Spiritual Foundations

In whatever part of the world you may find yourself, acknowledge as much as possible the cultural, indigenous spiritual foundations you are standing upon, geographically speaking. Acknowledge the specific indigenous techniques and attributes of prayer that are particular to the area, be they Native American, Maori, Vodun, Icelandic, Aboriginal, etc.

Step 4: Calling in the Spiritual Assistants

Now you can get on with it by calling in the power and authority of the world of spirit. You can call in the spiritual assistants, those out there in the spiritual realm, to come down and assist your prayer work.

As you reach up to the realm of the spiritual aides to support you in your prayer, you may ask them to come down and assist you. They may authorize you with some power and authority, or they may assist in or accomplish the task of the prayer. If you do this in a good way and with a good heart, then the chances are more likely than not that you may receive some spiritual intervention.

When calling in the spiritual assistants, the more specific you are, the better the possible outcome. What is the objective of your prayer? Why do you want them to come? What is their assignment, their purpose? What do you want them to assist you in accomplishing? How long are you asking them for their assistance?

It is important to specify all of this. Absolutely lay it out on the table, beyond a shadow of a doubt, maybe use spoken word.

Prayer for Healing

Here is an illustration of this. Let us say a woman is having a problem with her ovaries and asks you to help. Your petition to the spiritual assistants might go something like this: "I call on the spiritual doctors, as long as they have no ill will or malevolent intent, to assist me in my prayer of healing, for the time that this light being (the woman) is in front of me, assist me in the healing work of her ovaries. Your job is to help me fix these ovaries and bring them back to the feeling of balance and harmony again."

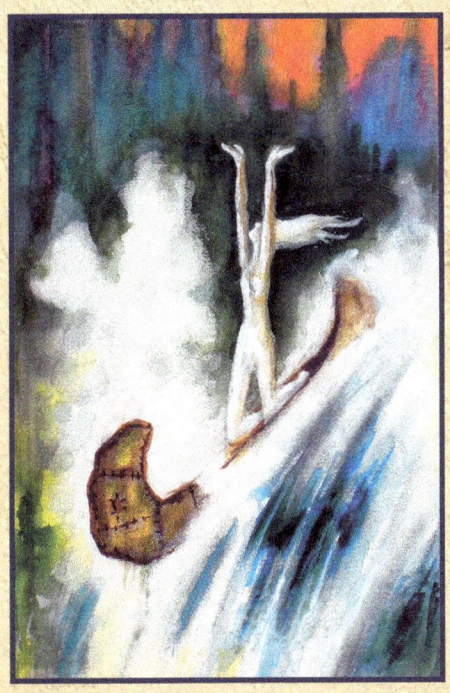

She Prays in Spirit

In praying in this specific way, you delineate the time factor, since you have specified that you are asking for help for the time that you sit and do these prayers. That means that when you are done doing these prayers, the spiritual doctors and spiritual assistants can return to where they came from.

Specify the time and the place, in a detailed manner.

When you specify that there be no ill will or malevolent intent, you limit the doorway between spirit world and our world. It is not good to open the door to the world of spirit without structure and knowledge. On the other side of that door there are many types. Who are they? Why are they there waiting? What do they want of this world?

There are good spirits and there are bad spirits. This is the natural order of the universe. It is one of the Universal Truths. It is important to be both aware and cautious of this, not to the point of paranoia but to a place of reason. So caution is recommended.

There are no guarantees in the spiritual realm just because you ask for something. However, the way you ask has great merit. The potential to manifest something is a whole lot stronger when done in a good way and with a good heart.

View spiritual matters as you view computers.[43] When you give the computer a complex calculation, it will give you an answer in a split second; as long as somebody plugged in the keyboard and input the necessary data to tell the computer what to do.

So in Spirit, one way of getting things done in good order is to put it all out on the table at one time: who, what, when, why, where and for how long. Everything seems to go more smoothly this way.

Step 5: Pray Hard

Pray hard. How long is relative to individual needs. You may set aside silent time with an alarm.

---

[43] This is not meant to be taken literally, but is an abstract concept.

Step 6: To Take ~ To Give Back

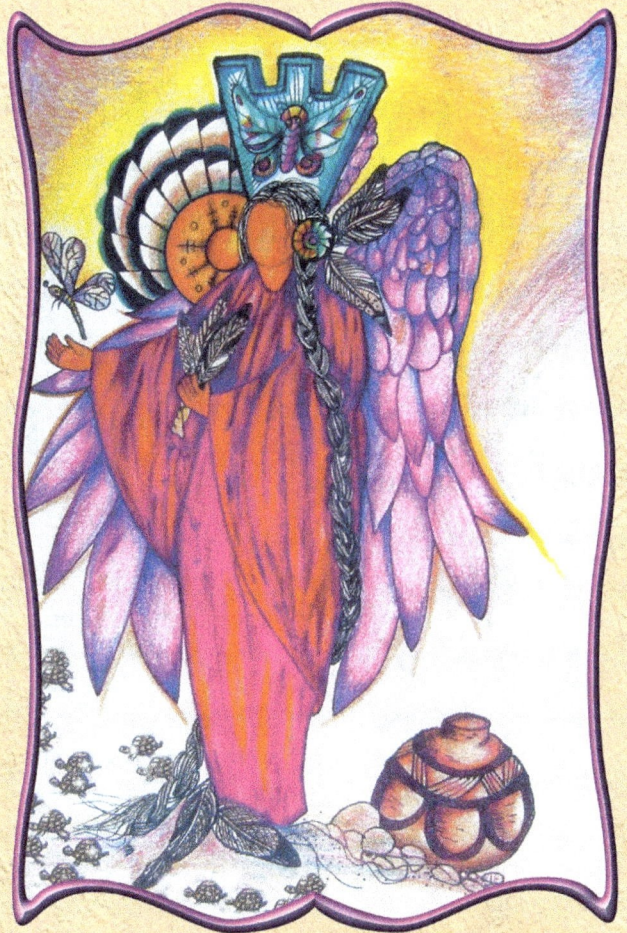

Angel With Purple Wings

Do not forget to complete the circle! When you have asked for something via prayer and you get what you asked for, be sure to say "Thank You." By saying this, you complete the circle in the form of an acknowledgment. This is not the only form of payment rendered.

This is a Universal Truth and here is a big difference between Native peoples and non-native peoples. In non-native society, things tend to be viewed as linear. One end of the line is Earth, our Mother, our provider, and at the other end of the line is the people.

People are good receivers, but at times can be not so good at returning. For example, look at how fast foods are becoming the dominant food source. After a meal, what is 'left over' is returned to the Earth, a big pile of plastic containers that do not biodegrade for centuries. We all have choices?

There is only so much Earth then there is no more. Well, the solution is so simple. The circle is the answer. To know and live by the concept that we are all related, "all my relations", can provide the solution if only taken to heart. It takes into consideration the effect of our actions not only here and now but also on generations to come.

We do not have an endless pocketbook at the expense of all our relations. We are all one. This is knowledge that Native Americans and other indigenous peoples can contribute to our future in a good way. What we do now effects the unborn.

We, as Two Legged People, do not have the right to discriminate about the power of prayer, because the power of prayer is universal. So you can pray for your mother that is ill, you can pray for your brother or sister who are ill, you can pray for yourself that is ill or out of balance, you can pray for whatever it is that you need. Again, be aware and avoid greed; keep everything in proportion in order to enable assistance with your prayers.

It's simple, just do it with a good heart in a good way.

FOOD

Food as a concept is universal and applicable to the other concepts about prayer. At our most important ceremony, we go without food and water for two days. On the third day, a small amount of sustenance is provided to the participants: two choke cherries, a teaspoon of buffalo meat and a half sip of juice. For many moons prior to the ceremony, this food is prayed for to charge it spiritually, beyond its protein and nutritional value. This charging comes by way of prayer, commitment, Will and Manifestation.

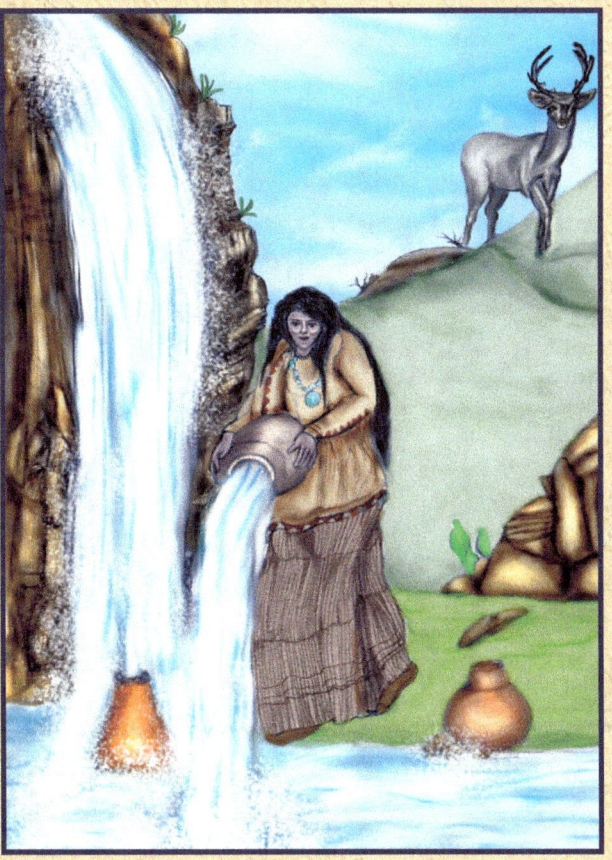

Give Away

Although we eat a small amount of food and receive its nutritional value, we also receive into this sacrifice of the foods' life, so that we as Two Leggeds may enjoy the value and honor that exchange.

Once adopted, the simple concept of praying over food to charge it spiritually as well as nutritionally and honoring the source from where it derives can become powerful tools in everyday life and survival into the future.

The linear world starts from the earth and goes to the people. However, the circular world starts from Mother Earth, goes to the people, and through the people's acknowledgment of its value and intent, goes back to Mother Earth.

This concept of balance is just like a circle, with no beginning and no end. This whole process is yet another cycle ~ the Natural Order of the Universe.

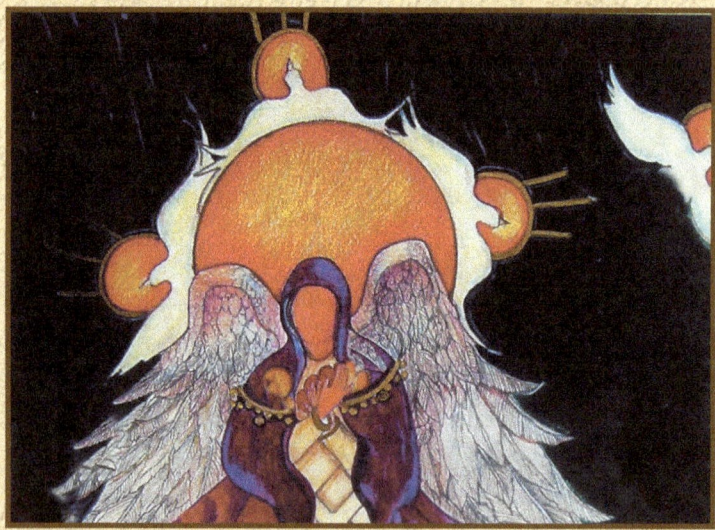

Angel With Sun

PRAYER AND CEREMONY

Prayer and ceremony are directly linked in our traditional way. Sacrifice is an affiliation of the present to the past. Some may say we don't have to suffer any more. Generally speaking, the Native American belief is to honor those who have given the ultimate sacrifice of their lives, for us now.

In giving our sacrifices we connect. Through sacrifice, we have the blessing of getting glimpses of what they, the warriors, women, little ones and elders have endured so that we could be here as free people, relatively speaking. Through this connection, we use prayer as a vehicle to achieve this ceremonial goal, freedom is one's 'right.'

With sacrifice, deprivation, ceremony, honor and prayer, we have an anchor to commitment, something that I view as severely lacking in most modern non-indigenous societies.

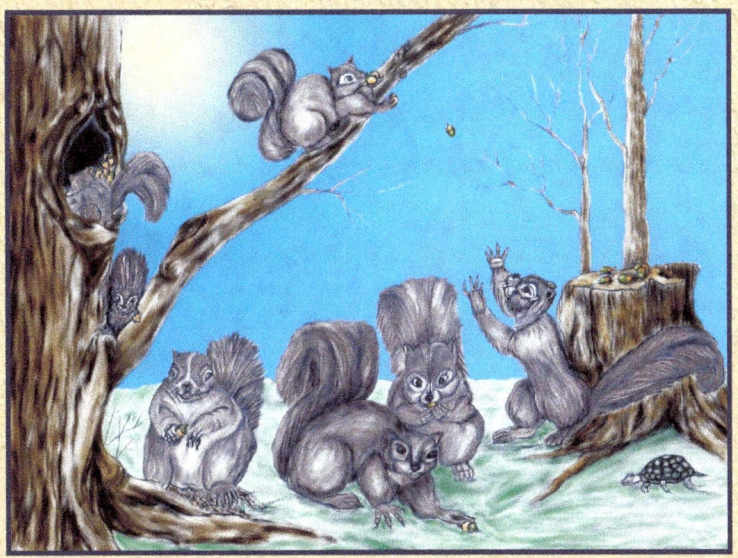

Gathering

TROUBLE

Here is where some people get themselves into trouble. They ask a bad person to put bad JuJu on someone, like a curse. The initiator of this is as responsible as the one who makes the curse. One thing most people do not realize is that by paying some bad-charactered person to do something, the initiator becomes deeply involved. They are far from being let off the spiritual hook. This weight is heavy; the payment for these kinds of spiritual debts will be far beyond the realm of dollars and cents. And if the price is not established beforehand, then when the initiator receives the results of those bad-intentioned prayers, they will be at the mercy of the greedy giver (and sometimes a greedy spirit) who will demand whatever price they see fit.

When it comes to this type of bargain, you can be sure that the price will far outweigh the goods received.

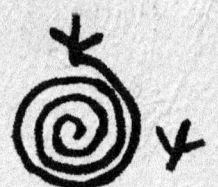

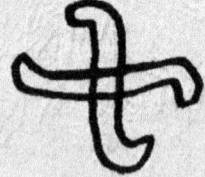

PRAYER AND BLESSINGS

In the Native American world there are many forms of bestowing blessings. Eagle feathers figure a lot in our ceremonies and prayers. Eagle medicine represents new beginnings, truth, and the messenger, which means anything having to do with messages, receiving them, giving or carrying them, etc.

One such practice comes from a southwest Tribal System in the United States. This is also a good example of the use of animals in blessings. The practice is to use some sort of natural material, like a local grass or sinew from an animal, to attach three[44] hummingbird feathers to the end of a stick that fits comfortably in the hand. The tips of the three feathers are then dipped in holy water.[45] The person giving the blessing is usually a person of stature or authority; they sprinkle the water on the one/s receiving the blessing, which could be a person or thing.[46]

Holy Water in this light can be considered a neutral substance. Of course, it is not neutral but for the sake of this teaching we will consider it so. As most of us are aware, numerous studies have shown the effects of an outside stimulus on water. For example, soft gentle instrumental music was played over a container of water. When the water was microscopically examined, it was revealed that its basic crystalline structure had been altered. When hard rock or anarchic styles of music were introduced, the water's crystalline structure was altered in a different way.[47]

---

[44] Regarding the use of sacred numbers in Native American culture, this is a reference to the three aspects of Two Leggeds: mind, body and spirit.
[45] Water that has been given a blessing by a medicine person, spiritual leader, Chief or someone of similar authority.
[46] "Thing" meaning an inanimate object like a necklace, ring, etc.
[47] Masaru Emoto has published several books that contain photographs of water crystals changed by "words of intent."

So here is an in-depth view of the function of prayer, the mechanics if you will. When a spiritual leader or holy person does a prayer over water, the structure of the water is likewise altered, this time in a spiritual way. This demonstrates the power of prayer.

People of faith understand this clearly, though sometimes in an indirect way. It's like being right but for the wrong reasons, but what of it? The reasons are immaterial! As long as the concept is there then so is the power. Will & Manifestation.

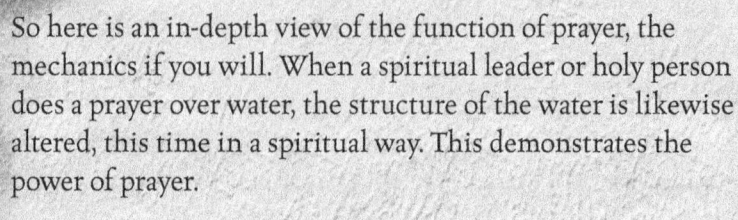

TWO LANGUAGES

A Two Feather concept: there are basically two languages,[48] one of faith, and one of science. Ok, let's give atheists a possible 3rd language, though they basically fall into the second category.

As light workers, the more we can corroborate spiritual matters with scientific matters the better. People of faith can use the language of science—statistics, demographics, charts, graphs, repeatable experiments, data gathering, and so on—to bridge the gaps.[49] The closer we get to world peace and greater understanding, the closer we get to Universal Truths.

The gap can be wide for sure. In some cases, there are those who point their fingers in a condescending way. It's easier to be negative than to come up with solutions. It requires expansive thinking and they tend to limit their higher aspects of thought. This is a form of self-sabotage. It's important that we, as people of faith, reach them, too, and I am saying that prayer is another way to do this.

To begin to bring about world peace, let us all build upon our similarities, work together toward common goals and understandings, and foster brotherhood, sisterhood and tolerance. Here there is an opportunity where Universal Teachings have a great value to serve us all, 'all our relations." The difference between the two languages is indicative of the separations that foster dysfunction of the highest good for all people. As individuals our voices, our actions, and our choices of how to live our lives are the ripples that reach out in their own way to all our relations.

---

[48] Regardless of the language, culture or color of the people, this is universal.
[49] In Book of Spirit, Vol. 3, Doctoring, this approach is explained in detail using examples of replicable methodologies and means of measurements that are acceptable to scientific communities throughout the world.

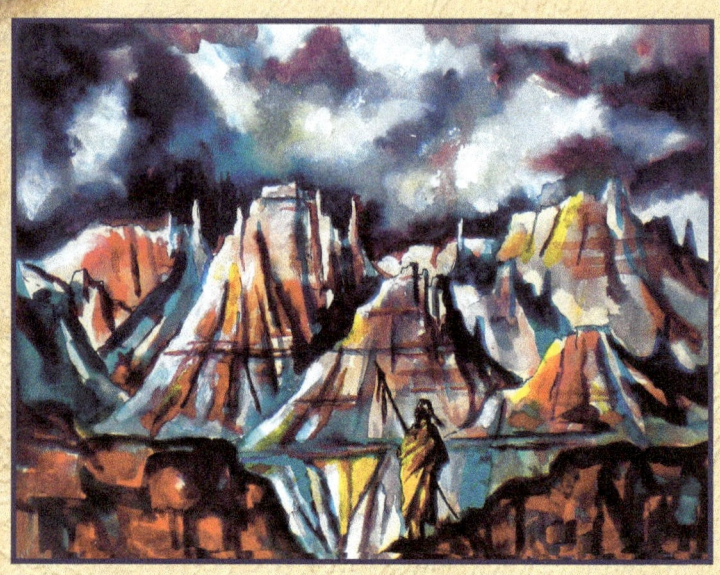

Warrior on Lake

What if you were this warrior standing alone at the edge of the lake? Can you go there in your powerful imagination? Ask yourself this: "what is important" to you. Now in your times of want or need, you can some here if you like. Aho.

SACRED CEREMONIES
Opening The Circle

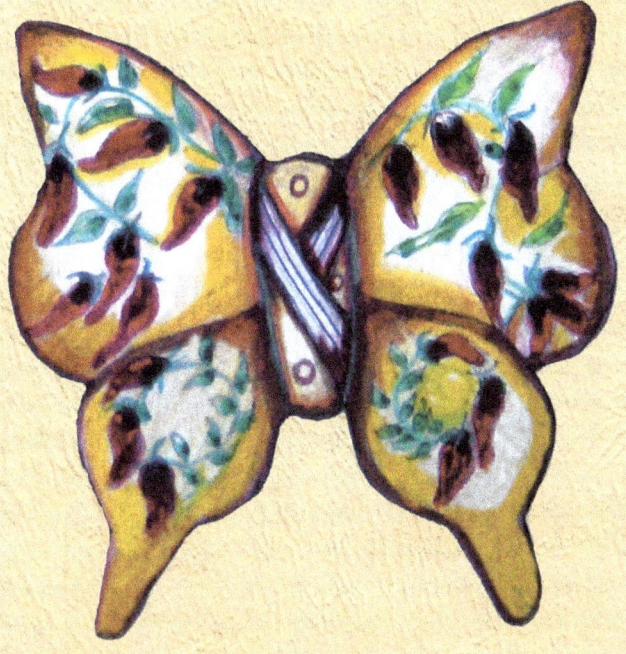

Butterfly

How to open a circle to pray in: face the direction that is appropriate to the petition/request you will be praying for.

* **The East:** new beginnings, babies born, seeds planted, the messenger, the color yellow
* **The South:** youth and vitality, bravery, protection, the color red
* **The West:** purification, bountiful harvests, introspection, young elders, healing, slowing down of life, the color black
* **The North:** wisdom, knowledge, spirit, respect, fulfillment, the place of long white hair, the color white

Face the direction that is most appropriate and find a place where you are least likely to be disturbed.

Locate a small rock or strong twig (give thanks) to scratch the earth with.

Smudge yourself with sage smoke for purification.

Set your intention. This is usually done silently, but if you feel yourself wanting to do otherwise, then do it. That's your own medicine kicking in. Just go with it.

Start to mark the circle in the East where the sun comes up and the day begins. Make a circle by moving your rock or stick clockwise along the ground. Once your hand is behind your back, transfer the rock or stick to your other hand, careful that the rock or stick does not break contact with the ground, as you continue to make your sacred area by moving it clockwise to complete your circle.

Smudge the circle with sage.

Call in protection, spiritual assistants, etc., as described earlier.

Then pray hard. Minimum recommended time for this type of prayer is twelve minutes. Thirty minutes is not out of range. Some people choose to pray for hours; it's relative to your individual needs.

Once you have used this medicine wheel, an imprint of your medicine is there. It should be closely guarded and kept out of harms way. Some elders say if you leave the medicine wheel unattended, you could be an easy mark for a bad person/spirit who could take your medicine as their own.

So be sure to close the circle[50] when you are done by using your hand to erase it counterclockwise (this is 'heyoka' or contrary.)

Be sure to leave an offering[51] to the Earth Mother you sat upon and scratched. Be mindful of the circle way of existence.

Talking Circle

The concept here is "community." If a problem is brewing in a community, the Talking Circle can help defuse it before it grows to proportions that are disruptive or detrimental to everyone, within that community

A leader calls for a talking circle and the word is passed along person by person—we call this "the moccasin express."

The ones who have been guided to join this ceremony sit in a circle upon the Earth, our Mother, usually around sundown, though it can happen at any time. The leader is the first to speak, laying out the agenda and structure for the Talking Circle.

Then the first person in the circle to speak their peace on the subject at hand is given the Talking Stick. Made by a creative leader in the community, the Talking Stick can be elaborately decorated or it can be plain, but it must have some appropriate symbolism on it.

---

[50] When done, one must close a circle once it has been opened. In this circle, you have opened your spirit; it is not wise to leave such a part of yourself without a respectful closing, as your individual medicine is within it until the one who opened the circle closes it. It is recommended that you do this yourself and not leave such a task to another!

[51] Appropriate offerings: a strand of your hair, not a glob, just one strand, as this is a witness of your spirit; a bit of saliva in a respectful way; something that you made with your own hands.

Whoever holds the Talking Stick is the only one permitted to speak. The leader should be gentle but authoritative on this point. A request is put out to please be respectful of others and not "hog" the time in an obtrusive way. Inevitably there will be one in the bunch who does not comply, but what can you say?

The Talking Stick is then passed from member to member, in a clockwise manner, until it goes around the circle one full time. This gives everyone a chance to speak uninterrupted. If someone breaks the circle by speaking out of turn, the leader will step in and do their duty to get things back on track, usually non-verbal, gestures work best.

The circle should not be broken once the ceremony has started; everyone should do their toilet thing before the circle begins. If someone has to leave the circle once things have started, they should ask permission from the leader in a non-verbal way. Usually, the leader will dismiss them from the circle non-verbally, by gesturing.

There is only one person in charge when it comes to this ceremony and that is the leader. Another time, another leader, that's fine. But once a leader is chosen or established for a ceremony, it's final. This leadership is critically important so that all who come have an opportunity to speak. Cohesion of community is a good thing.

After the circle is closed, everyone brings food and shares a meal together, even if it is one bite, for community.

The Talking Circle is a valuable mechanism that has been tested and used by many generations on Turtle Island.

Sweat Lodge

Another of the Native American People's sacred ceremonies is the Sweat Lodge. Sweat Lodge is considered our church for prayer, petition, purification, healing, and spiritual connection, by means of intense heat, steam, and sacrifice.

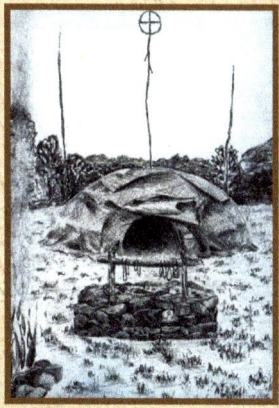

Sweat Lodge

The ceremonial area where this takes place is called the arbor. Within the area of the arbor, a roaring ceremonial fire is made and a lodge is built, a chest-high, dome-shaped structure made of bent over willow branches, covered with blankets or skins so the lodge is dark inside.

So small is the door leading into the lodge that the ceremonial participants have to enter on hands and knees, thus showing humility, while having as much contact with Mother Earth as possible and still being mobile enough to enter.

In the center of the lodge is the navel, a small pit where the dirt has been dug out. This dirt is then used to make a rectangular shaped altar, which is placed outside the lodge, two paces from the roaring fire[52], in the direction of the lodge door.

On the altar, the ceremony's participants place small items they want to be blessed. Usually there's a buffalo skull on the altar, too. The spiritual leader puts a special blessing on the altar items, as do the participants, in the form of prayer.

Rocks, aka Grandfathers, are made red-hot in the ceremonial fire and then brought into the lodge by the Fire Keeper, who

---

[52] Or one full stride, with one foot stationary and the other stepping as far as possible.

usually uses a long pitch fork. The Grandfather Rocks are then placed in the navel of the lodge.

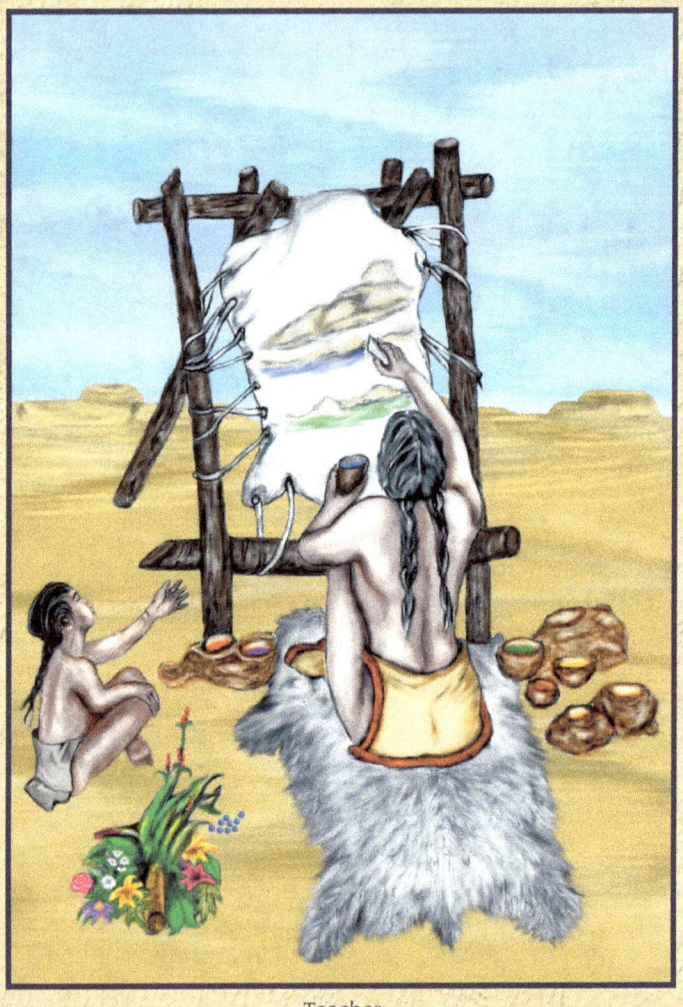

Teacher

This spiritual leader is also known as "the one who pours water" because he pours water over the Grandfathers and releases intense steam that lasts for many hours while we pray and tend to spiritual matters.

Only one who has given of their flesh and blood and had a

blessing from their O-ya'-te (spiritual leader) can be a leader. A male leader must have scars upon his chest, and a female leader must have strikes upon her arms or hands, as witness that they took part in a four-day ceremony with no food or water, when they were attached to the Cottonwood tree ~ the species of tree for ceremony.

For the hours[53] that the Sweat lodge ceremony takes place, many prayers are shared, in confidentiality.

There is a special connection between the ceremonial structure and the altar. They are designed so that the prayers go from the participants in the lodge, out the small door to the altar, through the eye sockets[54] of the buffalo skull (if there is one) and then finally up to Creator, who lives in the sky.

The ceremonial fire can also be a vehicle for prayer. This is considered sacred and the smoke helps carry the prayers to Creator, as it's lighter than air and rises.

Some people can say, "Well, that does not make sense."

Ok, it may not make sense from a western/scientific point of view, but the realm of spirit often defies reason and rationale.

It cannot be denied that prayer has function and structure, as do all other things in their own way. In most societies, the function and structure of prayer is present on the surface of the culture, or easily found within it.

Basically speaking, just as the structure of water is changed when prayers are done over it, so are the items on the altar changed when prayed over during Sweat Lodge. Their vibrational frequencies are altered; their base frequencies

---

[53] The heat and steam are intense. The shortest lodge I poured water for was about 2 ½ hours. The longest I can recall was about ten hours. The norm, if there is such a thing, is somewhere between four and six hours.
[54] It is common belief that the buffalo cannot see well on this Earthly plane but has vision into spirit world; therefore, the prayers are somewhat directed to the eye sockets to facilitate transference of the prayers to the other world we are petitioning to reach.

remain the same, but the items get a slight modification, a kind of "spiritual tune-up."

The strength of the effect depends on the faith of those involved. Consider malachite, for instance, a beautiful green stone with swirls. It is very soft on the Moe scale of hardness[55], but takes a good polish. The polish does not last long and the brilliance soon fades, relative to other harder stones. On the other end of the scale is ruby (corundum.) It's much harder and therefore holds a polish longer. The faith of the participants, the power and authenticity of the ceremony and the ceremonial leader, all these can be likened to the hardness of stones.

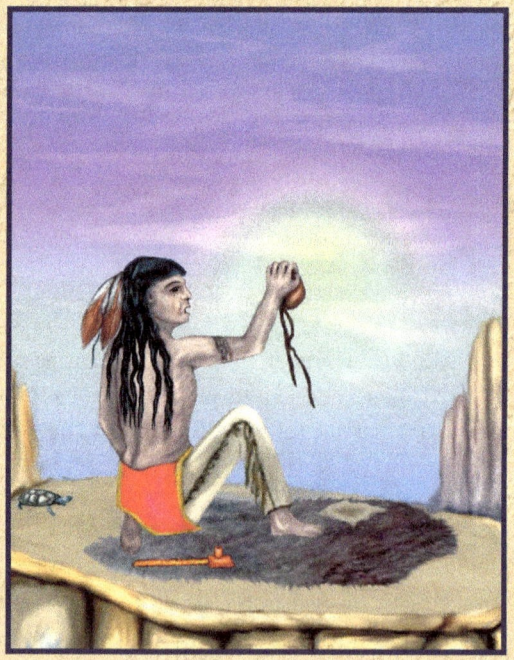

Prayer

---

[55] A standard scale used by gemmologists to determine the hardness factor of rock and gems.

PRAYER AS A VICTIM

Prayer can be a victim. For example, in the United States there is a law that says church and state are to be kept separate. So when there is a teaching in a public school with many hundreds of youth, if the presenter attempts to teach the group to pray, the presenter is then subject to penalties under the US law: fines, imprisonment, or both. In time, one gains enough experience to know to do the teaching in the form of asking in the traditional Native American way: 'with a good heart and in a good way.' To 'walk in beauty' is another old saying.

As we are made up of three essential aspects, how are these addressed in most of our public school systems in regard to our youth, our future?

Well, the physical aspect is dealt with in physical education. The mental aspect is addressed in memorization and testing. But what of our spiritual aspect?

Herein lies one of the truths as to why this series of books are being written ~ it is important to address our own spiritual life as well as well as the spiritual life of our youth. Shoving dogma down someone's throat just because it happens to be the accepted belief in a given geographical area is hardly conducive to fostering a cohesive society, nation, and world.

If, in our school systems, a general overview of many different belief systems and spiritual and religious teachings were made available, there would be much room for thought. People could take a heartfelt look and then subscribe to whatever they decide is best suited to their individual needs. Does our future lie in freedom of belief, tolerance and the ability to speak freely?

Our education system is due for an overhaul, and if we do not do it in a rational, systematic way, then what will become of our youth?

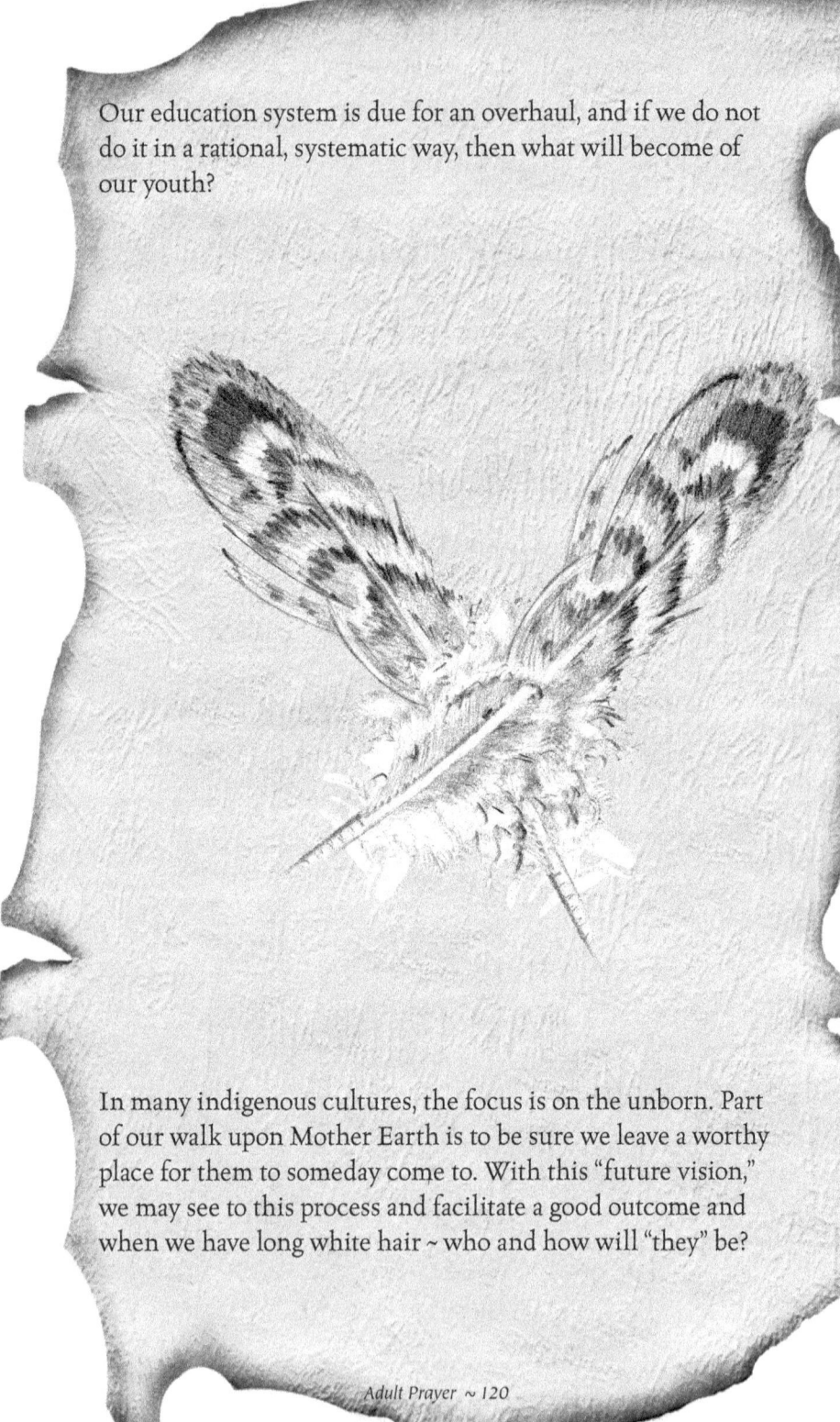

In many indigenous cultures, the focus is on the unborn. Part of our walk upon Mother Earth is to be sure we leave a worthy place for them to someday come to. With this "future vision," we may see to this process and facilitate a good outcome and when we have long white hair ~ who and how will "they" be?

PRAYER AND PRACTICAL APPLICATIONS
"The Hunt"

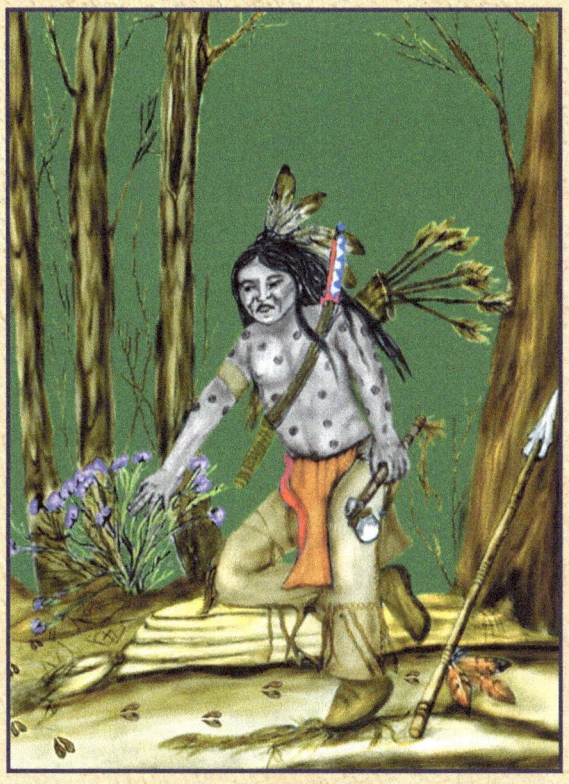

The Hunt

Some of these teachings are for stimulation of thought in a spiritually conscious light.

A long time ago, the Braves gathered for the hunt because meat storages were dwindling. Before the Braves left, they called for the services of a 'Hunting Medicine Person." [56] He

---

[56] Much effort has been taken to keep concepts and terminology discernible. Here, a better known term for this person would be "Shaman." This is not a Native American term but it is a Native American concept. For the duration of the teaching, this term will be used.

would accompany them to the place they knew was the best to find game, and then he would do his stuff. He was a respected component of that cohesive community with special skills. All gathered now to participate in the communal activity of hunting. This activity was reserved exclusively for males who had earned their place by merit.

The Hunt Shaman moved about, gathering certain plants[57] indigenous to that area. He found a special rock the size of two footballs that had numerous divots on it. Into the divots, he separated the plants until he had properly prepared them in the way he was trained by his teacher.

He burned some dried herbs, chosen for their medicinal qualities, to use the smoke. Then the Hunt Shaman prayed, making a chant he said over and over again. He was calling in the spirits, asking them to find the herd of deer and take the heart of the leader[58].

Once this had been accomplished, the heart was mystically brought to the Hunt Shaman.

The deer leader, with a great rack of horns, looked up immediately. He sensed that his heart was no longer inside him and knew what direction his heart was located in. Off he ran, followed by the herd as always.

By this time, the hunters were lying in wait, hiding between large boulders at a strategically favorable spot. The signal was given,[59] is honoured, and the hunters let loose until the pre-designated number of deers were downed. The leader is not taken. The hunter specialist returned the heart.

When the hunters returned, the village was happy and the

---

[57] It cannot be told what plants specifically, but I can say they are very colorful!
[58] Speaking of hearts, one of my teachers had been made aware of a dear, um, friend who had recently had a heart by-pass for the third time. Then is was no more hole.
[59] A particular animal sound.

women set about doing their important part in the survival of their community.

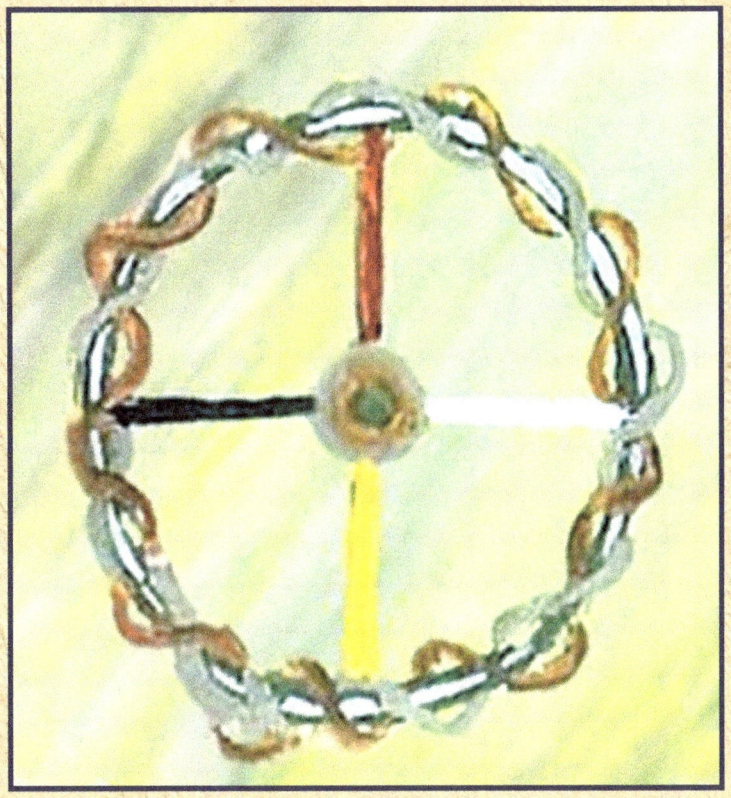

Medicine Wheel

It is mostly womans' work to prepare the meat, skins and meal. It was a rough way, but a good way.

Family and community were of great, great importance. The whole was the main consideration. Much has changed and we pray for that remembrance.

LIVING IN HARMONY WITH OUR ENVIRONMENT

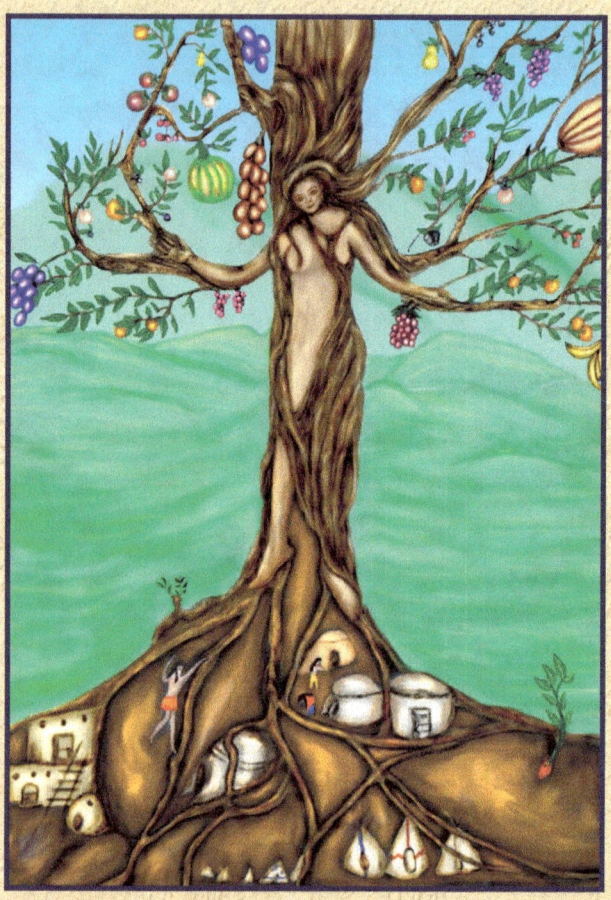

Tree of Life

W hy is it that the Native American people are viewed as living in harmony with the environment? One reason is that history shows how our ancestors stood still, watching the animals and the plants, and saw with more than just their retinas, irises and corneas; they listened with more than their eardrums, cochlea and auditory nerves. They learned and received much by being still and observant.

This has been passed down to us, too, for our development and growth, if we care to pay attention. We also have the innate abilities of universal hearing and universal sight. However, just as a person who lies in a hospital bed for weeks witnesses their muscles becoming droopy (atrophy) due to inactivity, so can our senses atrophy due to inactivity. Why use them when we have telephones, televisions, games and gadgets? Is this a result of evolution or by design? I ask myself "Is this what is right?"

People are used to not relying on their own senses. It's important to re-remember and re-connect if the world is to survive in a good way. Some words come to mind: self reliance, sustainability and accountability.

This is one reason why this assignment has been given by the elders to put into writing the teachings that up to now have been handed down solely through oral tradition. People around the world can learn a lot from indigenous cultures. This is something that has been discovered while traveling extensively throughout the world as a healer, a teacher of Native American Cultural Ways, and a Spiritual Advisor.

When we look at the big picture, it is easy to see that as free people, we do have certain rights. I, for one, am a veteran of the military. Freedom is well understood by us. We believe that it is our right to speak as we see fit, without fear that 'the powers' would only allow us to use their words and beliefs, or be punished or labeled. We should believe in ourselves by seeking knowledge.

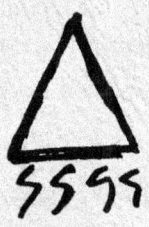

TOOLS TO AID PRAYER

Tools can provide extra power for prayer. Here is an example: into your mix of methods, add an abalone shell, perhaps as a place to burn herbs. It might not be so obvious but this is a way to bring in the blessing of the water people, since this is where the abalone shell came from, even more so if the shell was gathered in a way that completed the circle. If it wasn't, make your own offering anyway. It will help.

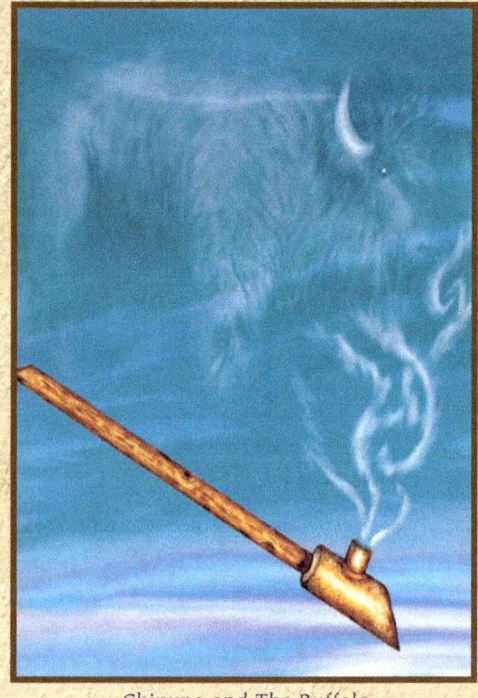

Chinupa and The Buffalo

Prayers administered by acknowledging and invoking, giving respect, gratitude and honoring, there is great power and authority here. To avail yourself of this can bring forth great mystery, to be used in the light, on behalf of those who are yet to come to the Earth and all others, including spirits in waiting. They deserve a decent place to come to. Just one person can make a difference.

We must consider the impact of our decisions on generations to come and prayer is one way to accomplish this. Set the Will and Intention, then just do it. You can be the one who calls the shots.

METHODS OF PRAYER
The Prayer Tree

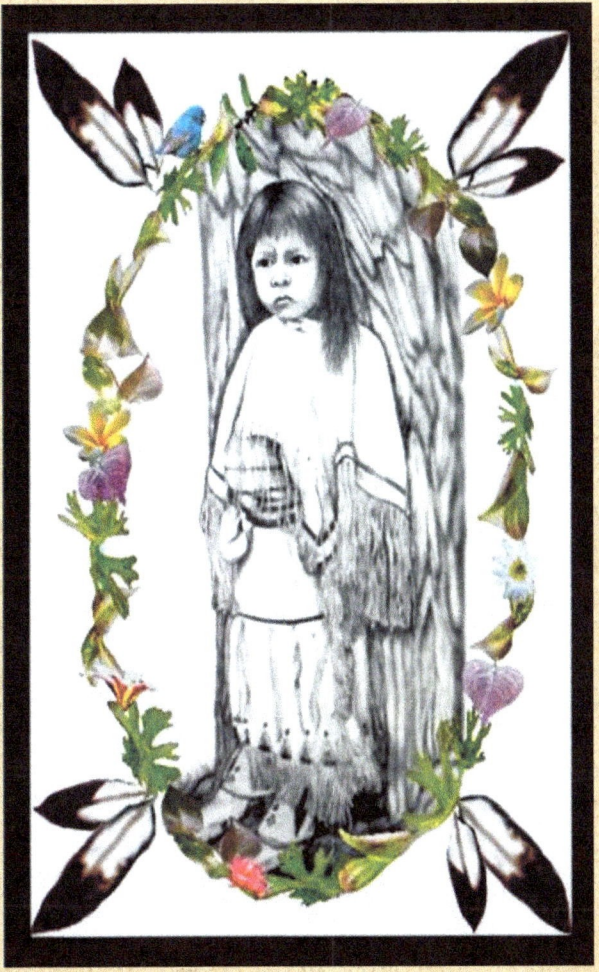

Apache Boy at Tree

A prayer tree is a One Legged Person (tree) with feathers tied on them. Each feather has had a prayer put into it and was then hung on the tree. The feathers act as an instrument between the prayer, the tree and Creator.

The spirit of the One Legged Person assists in holding and sending the prayers to Creator, just as the smoke did in the Sweat Lodge Ceremony. As time goes on, the tree grows bigger, carrying the prayers up closer to Creator. People who left prayers in the tree can come back to visit and see how high their prayers have grown.

It's been nice seeing more and more prayer trees going up around the world. You could start a prayer tree.

To make a prayer tree, you will want to gather a few items: a spool of strong twine and some feathers. Why feathers? The feather represents the wing of the messenger. There are two feathers that are not recommended: black colored feathers or owl feathers. All other feathers will do fine.

Now you are ready to find the One Legged Person. Be sure to consult the spirit of the tree before assuming it is OK. Going to ask them four times is a good rule. If permission is granted by the One Legged Person, you can go to the next step.

Surround the healing circle with white light. Inside the circle, fill it with cobalt blue. Call in the power and authority of cobalt blue to fill it with protection for the time you are doing this ceremony.

Most people prefer cobalt blue. Personally, I call in the color green for it represents Earth, our Mother. I call upon all her power and authority, and her protection from any one or any thing that has ill will or malevolent intent.

Now, hold a feather and be respectful. Make a prayer for what you want, and as you put that prayer into the feather, be specific. What do you want? What's the time frame? And anything else you think may be relevant. This is the power of prayer at work for you and that which you hold close.

Then tie the feather to a branch of the One Legged using a

piece of twine. Tie it loosely to allow for tree growth, but make a strong knot, though not necessarily thick[60].

People get caught up in technique. It's really not as important as the underlying concept. Your medicine is far stronger than mine, so just let it flow. Some may make mistakes and be bigger for it and grow.

If the proper intent is put into practice, it will all work out. In a good way and with a good heart.

The making of prayer trees around the world is one of the platforms of Native American Spiritual Prod. (N.A.S.P.)

The objective of N.A.S.P. is to bring together indigenous healers, teachers and spiritual leaders from around the world to share their well-intentioned ways with others.

N.A.S.P. supports three basic concepts: World Peace, the Unification of All Nations, and Responsibility for the Unborn ('unborn' meaning the spirits who have yet to come to Earth. We are the ones who are responsible to see to it that they have a worthy place to come to.) Also, to keep this in our hearts and ways "future by design."

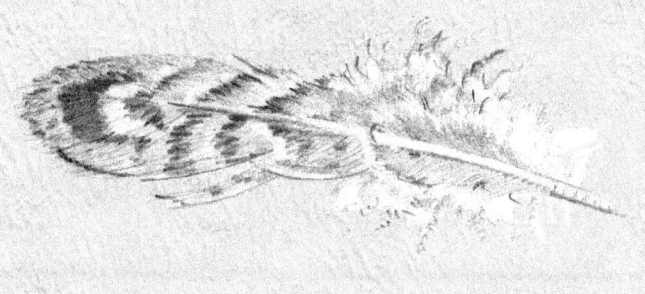

---

[60] Make an effort not to hang the feathers too low; in the past (rarely) the dark side has been known to come in the darkness of night and, in evilness, cowardly steal all the prayers.

Group Prayer

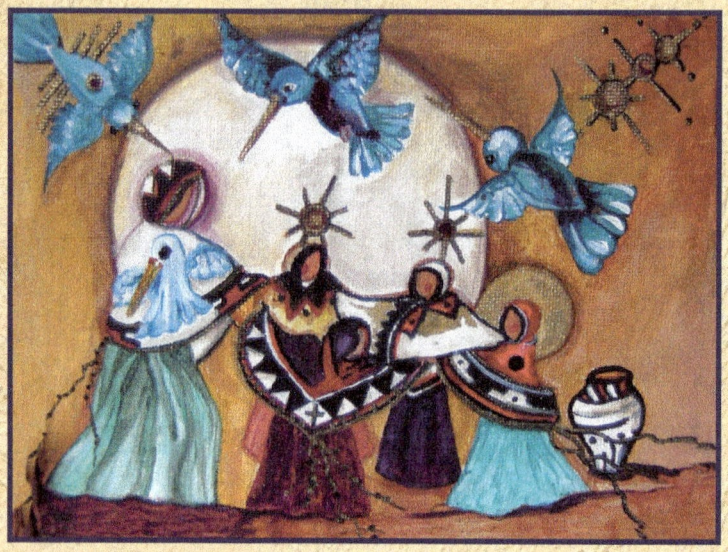

Hummingbirds

It is often customary, or simply more beneficial, to work prayer in a group. The more energy that is involved, the more connection there is to spirit, and the more powerful the effect.

For example, in a Southwest tribal system on Turtle Island we do a rain dance. It is done in the shape of a fan. One dancer stomps his feet in a prescribed manner accompanied by a specific drumbeat. Consider the slapping of a hand in a calm pool of water: the results are ripples. So is it with stomping feet. Add another stomping person to the first, then add ten more, then thirty more. This builds an ever-growing vibrational frequency that spirals upward and outward. Along with a few other good things[61], there comes rain.

I have also seen a weather shaman put his fingertips into a lake to make rain. Doing so in a good way and with a good heart represents the mastering of the art of prayer. It can be

---

[61] Go figure?

done! Elements are here to serve man or is it the other way around?

Prayer Ties

Here is another ceremonial way of praying; an established, community-supporting means of spiritual interaction. The objective is to put your prayers into tobacco and join them with the prayers of the community onto a series of four strands of prayer ties that will be burned, allowing the prayers to be released and carried by the rising smoke up to Creator.

What more of a blessing could there be, short of an eagle flying over-head and taking the prayers into her talons and then flying them herself up to Creator?

To make prayer ties, you will want to get a few things:

* Tobacco. The most popular brand is American Spirit, all natural; the only brand frowned upon is "Red Man."
* A lot of string, about half the thickness of shoestring.
* Four large pieces of cotton cloth, each a color representing one of the four directions: yellow, red, black and white. Cut the cloth into two-inch squares. Have enough for everyone to make at least one prayer[62] with. For thirty people, one large shopping bag full should do.

When possible[63], participants are advised to smudge with sage before entering the ceremonial area where prayer ties will be made.

---

[62] Participants are encouraged to make as many prayers as they care to. Gathering the necessary amounts of material should be dealt with prior to the ceremony. Ceremonial leaders are expected to delegate duties and to supervise so that everyone gets to participate if they want to.
[63] At some public functions it is forbidden to make fire, so you'll need to incorporate a little wolf medicine and come up with other ways to accomplish this. Can you smudge outside before entering the structure (if there is one.) Use a van, station-wagon or car?

Once you enter the area, sit in the direction that corresponds to what you are praying for: love, protection, healing, wisdom, etc. Place a pinch of tobacco in your hand and hold it up to the sky and pray ~ with pride and reverence. Usually the arm would extend upwards from a sitting position, since the most favorable results occur when the body is touching the Earth.

The medicine of the tobacco plant is retention of memory. So when you make a prayer while holding tobacco, the prayer will be stored inside, each little piece like a hologram.[64]

Next, choose a piece of colored cotton that corresponds to the direction your prayer relates to. Place the pinch of tobacco in the center of a cotton square. One way to do this is by placing the cotton square on the hand holding the tobacco and then carefully over-turning the hand.

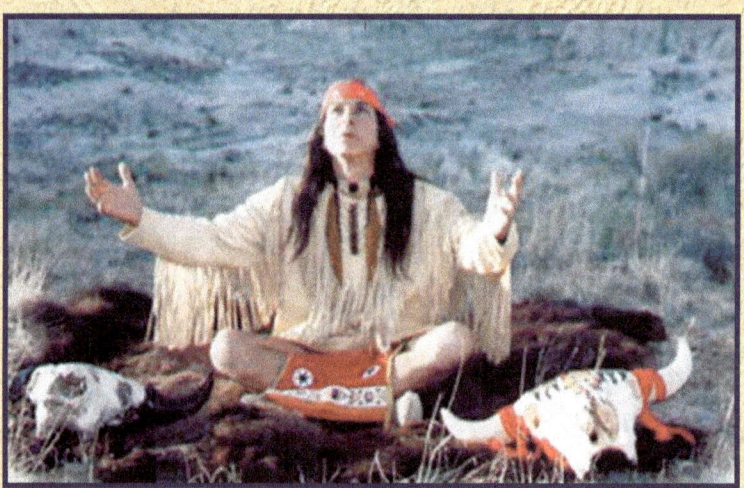

Praying For A Vision

Gather the ends of the cloth together while keeping the tobacco bunched in the center. Now wrap a piece of twine around the ends to tie them off, so the tobacco will stay snug

---

[64] I predict someday we will make an agreement with the tobacco plant people and tobacco will store memory for us, like a computer, though in a more expanded-consciousness way.

inside the newly formed prayer tie. I usually twist the string to the right, make a loop and pull it tight, and then twist to the left and make a half hitch knot. Give it a good tug to make sure it won't come unraveled.

When you are done, tie your prayer tie to one of the four strands that corresponds to that direction. So, for instance, all the red prayer ties would be tied on the same strand, all the black on another strand, etc.

Then step back from the prayer tie making area and permit others to have their time to make a prayer tie. Once everyone has made at least one, its open house for all to make as many as they feel compelled to do. Since only four people can sit in this area at once (one for each of the four directions) this will take as much time as necessary.

Try different directions for different types of prayers, if you feel guided, until your petitions are complete.

Once they are put on a string, prayer ties should not have any contact with the Earth, and should stay together. It is not good to break a string with prayer ties already on it. If this happens, please tie the string together as soon as possible. You will end up with four strands of as many prayers per strand as were made, for that was how many were supposed to be made.

It is good for the participants to bring a dish of food so that after the prayer ties have been made and put in a safe place, all gathered can share a meal. A small plate of the food is put together and left out all night, called a 'spirit plate.'

A trusted Keeper of the Prayer Ties (KOPT) is chosen to fulfill the destinies of the prayers and be responsible for keeping all four strands together for four days.[65] Each day in waiting is in

---

[65] Although this teaching is meant to be a guide, do something different if you feel compelled. It is your ceremony. Do good and all will be well.

honor of the Grandfathers and Grandmothers of each of the four directions.

At sundown on the fourth day, the KOPT builds a small sacred fire to finish the journey of the prayers. Kindling is piled in four separate heaps corresponding to the four directions. It's nice to say a small prayer when lighting the sacred fire. The East is usually lit first, then the South, the West, and lastly the North.

When the fire is strong, the prayer ties are put into it in a respectful way by the Keeper of the Prayer Ties. Follow the pattern of the circle. Stand in the East and put in the yellow prayer ties and release the prayers. Once the ties are in the smoke, go to the next direction, the South, and respectfully put in the red prayer ties, releasing them on their journey. Next is the West for the black prayer ties, and then the white prayer ties are placed in the North. The burning of the prayer ties on the fourth day into ashes and smoke releases the KOPT from their responsibilities and duties.

If possible, do not put any foreign objects in the fire; remember this is a sacred act. Sometimes things have to be changed for practical reasons, and that's OK. It's the Will and Manifestation that matters; the details of ceremony and ritual are guidelines and tools. Some situations may require you to improvise. For instance, fires may be banned in your area. In that case, a barbecue might come in handy if that kind of fire is permitted.

Be resourceful, use what is at hand, and let the ceremony happen. Sometimes we are asked to make sacrifices on behalf of accomplishing our prayers. Know that as long as you are pure of heart, you have nothing to fear ~ bullets cannot kill you and poison cannot harm you.

Other factors can be taken into consideration, like the

actual geographical location of the blessing/prayer. If it is a sacred site[66], long-standing ceremonial grounds, an energy wellspring, blessed area, lateral energy flow etc., your prayer will have the power of that energy with it. If there are animals in the area, they can also have an influence on the blessing, depending on the species, their intentions, physical condition, etc.

The plants and trees can also have some indirect effect (intervening variables.) If the area is surrounded with ancient trees like the Cowry[67] or Bristlecone[68], they will definitely have an effect on the prayers/blessings.

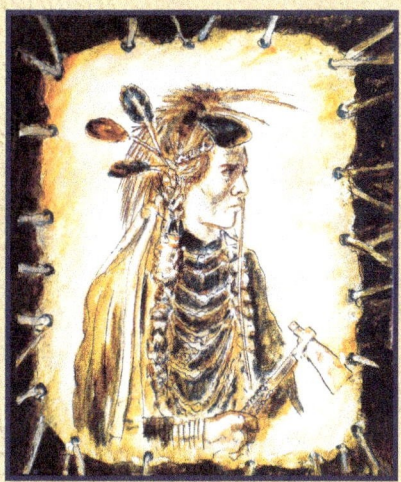

Warrior with Tomahawk

---

[66] An intersection of two ley lines that create anomalous Earth behaviors resulting in altered vibrational frequencies.
[67] Oldest trees in the world that I am familiar with. They live in northern New Zealand. I have had the purposeful adventure of going to visit them on occasion. What a blessing they are!
[68] Oldest trees in the western hemisphere that I am familiar with. They live in very few places. One is above my hometown of Taos, New Mexico, on the Enchanted Hwy. loop. Well worth the trip.

WE ARE ALL RELATED

In the final analysis, we are all related: "Mitake Oyasin", All My Relations. Each and everything around us is us, and thus deserves all the respect and consideration we would desire for ourselves.

Here is the crux of it all: we are the universe and the universe is us. What a different world it would be if we, all people (7 billion plus) subscribed to the Native American way, the way of the circle.

The circle has no beginning and no end, the circle "is."

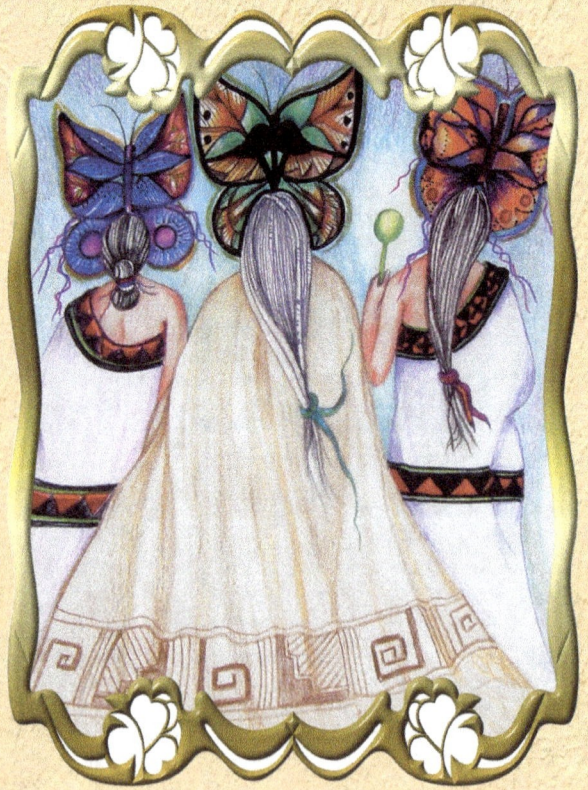

Butterfly Women

IN CONCLUSION

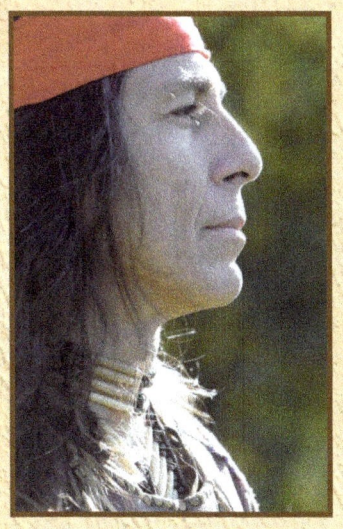

Two Feather

Now that you have had the opportunity to find your way through these written teachings that traditionally have been passed on orally, your psyche has been installed with tools that can serve you when the need arises. The psyche will rise to its purpose at the time and place that's appropriate. AHO.

Some of the concepts have been very deep, while others may seem, on the surface, so obvious. In the final analysis, your heart will lead the way. There within lies your key. Use it wisely.

For me it has been a long haul, over eleven years of dedicated and passionate writing. I can remember having a spoon of food in one hand while the other hand was on the keyboard, in the process of getting one more teaching down.

All the books in the series are written "for the people."

Inspiration has come from everywhere. A lot of the writing was done in Australia, hopping all over the country in six week increments. Other writing locations included the United States, the Orient and South America. What a blessing!

I say thank you to my parents, William Senior and Aurora; to my teachers; to all those who came to me for healings; and to all those who I have had the honor and pleasure of imparting some of this knowledge. Thank you to Rhonda, Dor, BB and the Texas crew who supported and had faith in this spiritual project. Bless you all.

There will be a total of 12 books in this series. These first five are just the beginning, I am sure of that.

I look forward to spending more time with you in the future as you become familiar with the way of My Native American People, within our culture - we are the Turtle Island People.

AHO ~ William Two Feather
Pray with a good heart and in a good way! Walk in beauty.

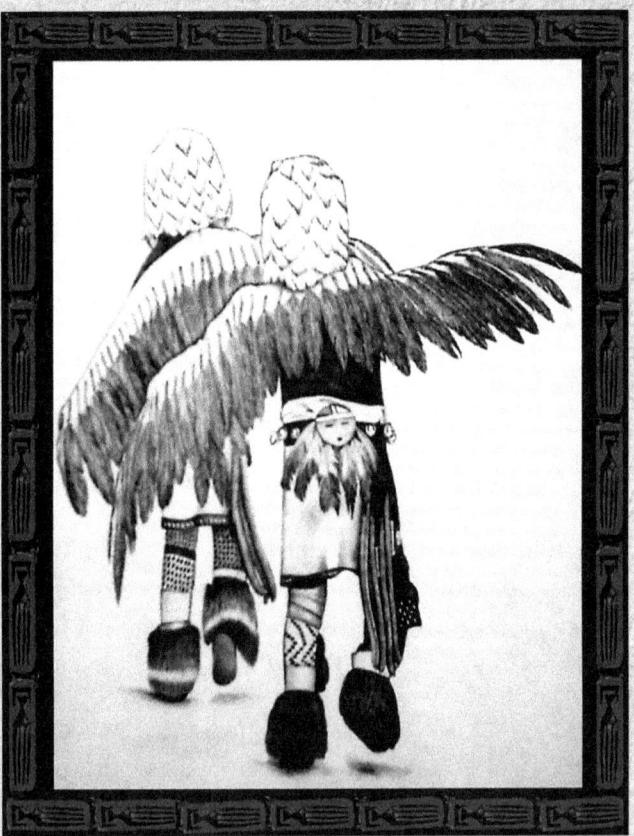

Eagle Dance Boy

ACKNOWLEDGEMENTS

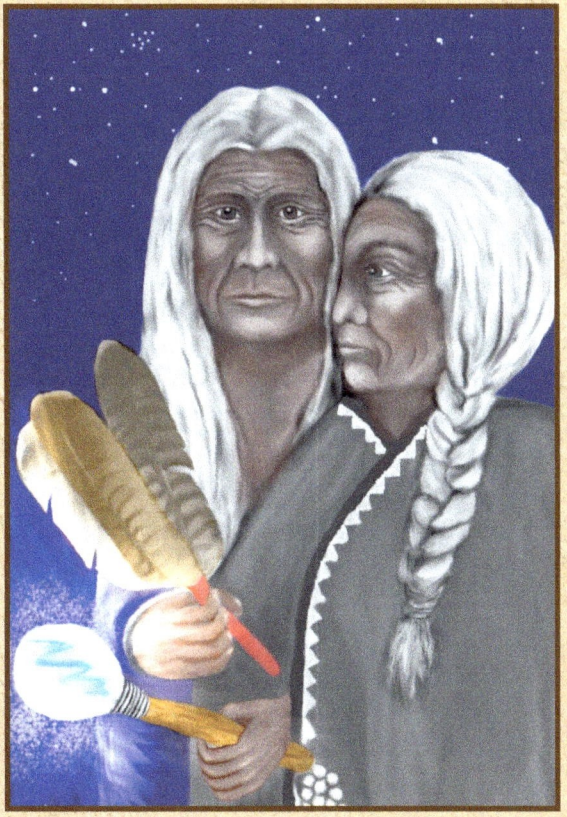

Oy Ya Te

The gratitude for those who contributed to the completion of this book is immense. Thanks to my mother Aurora and father William Senior, also to the artists; Beth of Australia, Paula of Albuquerque, New Mexico, Maria of Taos, New Mexico, USA, and Nicole of San Diego, California, USA. Much gratitude goes to the editors, especially Janice Terra (Lady Horse Whisperer) of Houston Texas and Tim Fried- Fiori. Thank you to Linda of Australia for your assistance.

A word of thanks to the Countries and those who contributed

knowledge from the elders and provided safe haven for the writings for over 11 years; Turtle Island USA, Costa Rica, Italy, Nicaragua, Australia, Dominican Republic, Japan, China, England, Slovenia, Greece, Wales, and Scotland.

Thanks many times over to my three teachers; Wind Walk, Grey Wolf, and Prays to the Morning Star. And those elders both Grandfathers and Grandmothers, healers and Spiritual leaders of many countries ~ may Creator bless you well for your sharing. Your positive re-enforcements felt like rocket fuel.

Many thanks to the people who provided safe haven for the nuts and bolts to be written; Linda Longa of Australia, the Tivoli Family and Linda of the Blue Mountains, Grandmother Gatekeeper, the people of Florida, Texas, Arizona, and New Mexico. Thank you to those who reside on tribal lands on Turtle Island USA. Thank you Jeff of Taos.

Thanks to those who provided inspiration on this project; Beth, Linda, Sue, Chloe, Bree, Chief Marvin Swallow, Mary of Thunder Ranch, Rhonda, Dawn, Janice, Diane, Nicole, Florance, Rev. Michael Beckwith of The Secret, and Basha of The Tokyo Museum. Much inspiration came from alternative healing centers and metaphysical conferences all over the world. Your patronage spurred me on to more writing. Thank you to Unity Center of Oslo Norway.

Thanks to the "Tough Love" wilderness camps, seeing their need for guidance and the wide-eyed joy they had in receiving wisdom, spurred me forward to taking pen in hand to write down the oral traditions while they are still here. For the youth yet to walk on Mother Earth, you are our inspiration. For you we honor, sacrifice, preserve and nurture. Thank you Schools of Waldorf.

A huge honouring goes to Spirit and those beings from the

light who had a hand in this process. So often when I felt like I was at the end of my reserves, a miraculous event would intervene to help guide me on. Thank you to those supporters who see to it that indigenous ways do not become a thing of the past. Thank you to the educational facilities, which encourage self-growth. We all have our paths to walk upon. The more knowledge we have access to, the greater we can be of service to others. To acknowledge is to complete the cycle ~ the circle ~ The Wave...........

Dhan Zhou, William Two Feather

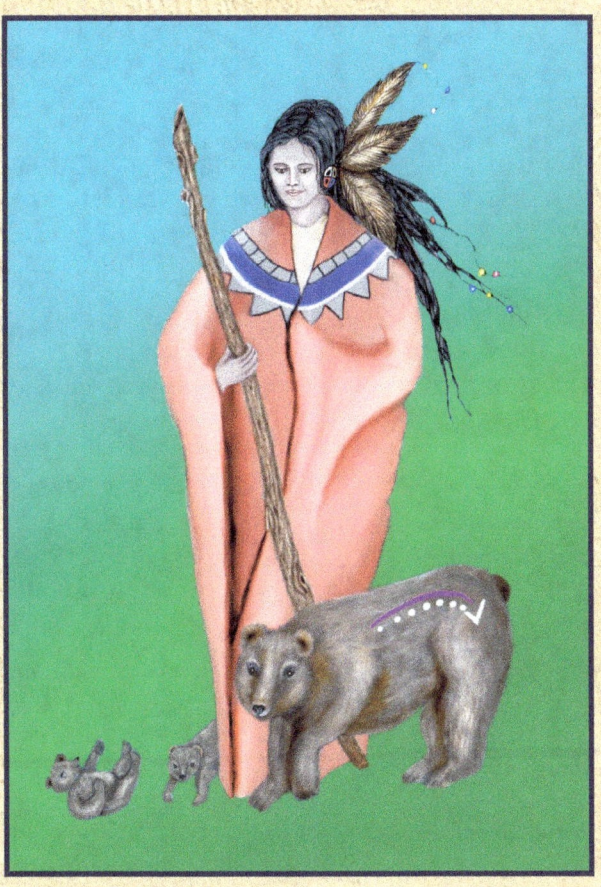

Matron Spirit Woman of The Bears

GLOSSARY

All Below (noun) ~ term commonly used in ceremony and prayer. That is the earth and all below. Most Indian tribes believe there are people living in the earth. Some believe one race and others believe several. The consensus is there are people living in the earth but they do not look like us and some are called the hideous. But to them we are.

Assessment (noun) ~ a visual appraisal of a client by watching the body language very carefully. Skeletal disorders are easy to spot with a visual assessment. Be aware of slowness or jerkiness of movement and favoring one side or part of the body. Facial expressions, eyes semi-closed, attune your sight to anything that doesn't seem right.

Count Coup (verb) ~ The first thought often conjured up when speaking of counting coup is the accumulation of the accolades of bravery and honor through scalping. But scalping was not an Indian thing; it was introduced by the invaders as a way of continuing the decimation of the First People, in order to take our land. The old way of counting coup was to take one strip of meat from the enemy you personally killed. The skin was then made supple

and attached to a war shirt. Could you imagine a young buck, with only two strips on his war shirt, rounding a tree to find a veteran warrior with 40 strips? Sometimes it's wiser to run away and live to fight another day, but I've not been able to practice that myself too much, oh well. The shirt is also referred to as a 'Ribbon Shirt'; nowadays, its strips are made of colorful cotton. Hmmm.

Dhan Zhou Apache for what do you need or salutation

Etheric Field (noun) ~ also known as aura, which is the electro-magnetic energy field surrounding the body. It has two layers, one that is about three to seven inches from the body and a second layer outside of the first that extends out to two feet. On average it extends about one and a half feet. Different people have different thickness, lengths, colors and strengths.

Fetish (noun) ~ a hand-carved item that sits near the top (closest to mouth) of the flute, usually carved in some animal image. This one was made from black and red corral and turquoise. The Zuni people of the southwest for well know for this.

Four Directions (noun) ~ North, South, East and West, each having it's own particular medicine. Respective of each other they are referred to as the work of Grandmothers and Grandfathers and they are the ones who hear petitions from those who seek or pray accordingly.

Grandmother (noun) ~ Metaphorical term meaning "woman" or female who has walked this earth many moons.

Grandfather (noun) ~ Same as above with long white hair except male or masculine.

Tomahawk (noun) ~ a hand held axe for war. Twin hawks means she threw two at a time and always hit the target.

Healing Tools (noun) ~ That which healers use to do their work. They can be made of animals, plants, stone, etc.

Light Worker (noun) ~ A person of any age or gender who is a warrior for what is right for all. Some are formally trained in "Spiritual Warrior Teachings" and some are of their own cloth and chose consciously or were drafted by who knows who ~ Spirit.

Medicine Person (noun) ~ One who is formally trained in medicine (healing) and given blessing by their teacher or spiritual leader. This position seems to have an opponent wanting to wear those moccasins, so this term is used in general context.

Medicine Wheel (noun) ~ In the shape of a circle depicting no beginning and no end. The medicine wheel always is the foundation of the Spiritual beliefs of many indigenous people. There are many different types of medicine wheels: for keeping time, healing, communal gatherings and seeking spiritual guidance, to mention just a few. In indigenous cultures, the approach is circular. When we receive something from Mother Earth, or a gift from a totem animal or spiritual assistant, we stop and acknowledge what we have received. This completes the circle. In this way, we acknowledge all our relations and honor our relationships to them. Indigenous people believe that this approach of 'completing the circle' could be a benefit to many if practiced in daily life.

Oyate (noun) ~ A spiritual leader of considerable background and reverence. In the Dakota language, the word for "people."

PA (noun) ~ (Personal Assistant)-team including a PA who's in charge of the other staff

Pipe Carrier (noun) ~ In order to be a pipe carrier, one must participate in a specific ceremony that requires months of preparation, four days of fasting, and sacrifices of flesh and blood. As I travel the world, people who have a Chinupa sometimes approach me, however these people have not participated in the required ceremony. They bring their pipes to me for a blessing and I do this, but I also restrict the use of the pipe to their selves only! Any other use, especially to satisfy the ego, is not permitted. The pipe is for the people, and times are changing, so we bend like the willow to survive and preserve the 'way of the pipe', given by Pte San Win, White Buffalo Calf Woman. Thank you all pipe carriers for your service to your communities!

Preparation (verb) ~ Appropriate in many places, the self, the client, the location, the tools, an object, your attire, etc. Paves the way for healing work. It is purposeful and focused on a particular petition.

Prime objective (noun) ~ To do the best job possible in serving each and every client, community or ceremony.

Relatively speaking (adjective) ~ Not absolute. Remember, things don't always make sense or are rational.

Rendezvous (noun) ~ A gathering of people for a weekend camp out returning to a turn of the century way of life when fur trappers first came to American Indian land. Many were honorable and lived in harmony with the other community members in a rough sense.

Rez (noun) ~ Short term for reservation, our own Indian land where we have sovereignty.

Self- healing (verb) ~ Ones innate ability to heal their own body, mind or spirit.

Smudging (verb) ~ Burning of dried herbs, roots or barks for the smoke to purify an area or client.

Specify (adjective) ~ May be done with one of the three powers of the word: Spoken, Written, Unspoken. A specific function with a target / goal, stated explicitly.

Sun-Dance (noun) ~ The highest of all Native American ceremonies, it occurs on the summer solstice, around June 21st. It includes four days of dancing in the circle for our Mother Earth, and we also make a petition of our own. I have attended for many years, honoring a commitment in this way. Sundancers must give flesh and blood each year. During the ceremony. Enough said about that.

Two-Legged (noun) ~ A typical way Native American people use to refer to different species is to delineate by the numbers of legs. Two-legged refers to humans, one-legged for trees and thick plants.

Will & Manifestation (noun) ~ Two terms of special gifts given by Creator, or intention and result.

Wind Walker (noun) ~ Term used for one who has died in this body, gone to Spirit and come back. He (my second teacher) has experienced two incidents that I know of when he was pronounced clinically dead.

We (adverb) ~ It is a rule of thumb to do healing work with an assistant always present for many reasons.

Zuni (Noun) ~ Southwestern tribe of Indigenous people known to be fine craftsman of inlaid silver jewelry.

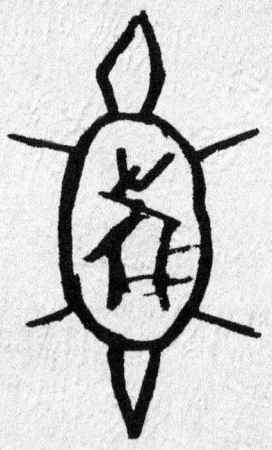

ART CREDITS

Page i   **The Power of Prayer / Epiphany**
Cover : Nicole Plaisted - Artist
Desert Sage San Diego, California, USA

The symbols in this drawing tie together many of the Native American Nations that make up Turtle Island. The first symbol is the large pink Lotus/ Apache symbol in the top center of the drawing. This represents the entry point for Spirit to come through and bring wisdom to the person who prays for that knowledge. The figure in the center represents the Universal stance of Prayer with arms upraised in gratitude and wonder at the Great Mystery and the answers that have come. Down the arms of the coat are symbols from the tribes of the North West. The base of the coat symbolizes the wave, which has been known to the people of Turtle Island as the energetic vibration or force that connects us all. To the right of the figure there is a pictograph drawing on the wall that is a representation of Hopi Prophecy Rock. The sky holds the mystery of the Animal Spirits The Eagle and The Buffalo who help to guide us on our journey. The Dolphins, or people of the sea, remind us that the wave is always present in a physical form as we watch how dolphins swim and play.

Page ii   **Two Feather**
Accompanying Spirits of a Feather original digital composition by Beth of Australia. Designed as a poster for one of the myriad of sayings developed by William Two Feather over a long writing career. The clever and cunning of the wolf and the looks with-in medicine of the bear have served the people in a way of assisting in healing and spiritual work.

Page iv   **Strength**
An appaloosa pulls a heavy load of rock people as a testimony to strength. Grandmother Maria of Taos, New Mexico,

original graphite, then colorized digitally in Australia by Beth of Melbourne. The zia at top represents the state flag of New Mexico, USA and the petroglyphs on the rocks being pulled is that of history, being carried on into the future.

Page 4   Elders
Elders representing the four directions. In the bottom left is an Eskimo Grandmother. Top left is Geronimo, top right a Spiritual Leaders from the north and east, bottom right is Two Feather Spiritual Advisor. Grandmother Maria of Taos, New Mexico, originally graphite, then colorized digitally in Australia by Beth of Melbourne.

Page 5   Lovers
She has been waiting patiently. Digitally graphically rendered by Beth of Melbourne, Australia. The colors flow in the light of love.

Page 9   Mystery
What is inside the cave? What's outside the cave? What's going on here, why is there a comet in the sky, and why is there a fire on the Plateau? Grandmother Maria of Taos, New Mexico, original graphite, then colorized digitally in Australia by Beth of Melbourne.

Page 10   The Apache Woman
Stands next to world renowned basketry, and some pottery. The long fringe on her shirt represents southwest Apache. Paula Manning of Albuquerque, New Mexico and Feathered Frame by Beth of Australia.

Page 11   Babushka
The Russian representative of woman's rights sacrificed herself for the good of woman's suffrage and the equality to vote and have equal rights to men back in the old days. Photo courtesy of Jasna Kovac of Kopper, Slovenia.

Page 14   **Transformation**
Grandmother Maria of Taos, New Mexico, USA, original
graphite, then colorized digitally in Australia by Beth of
Melbourne.

Page 15   **Spiritual Warrior**
She floats in the clouds two mighty Hawk Feathers in her
hand ~ prepared for spiritual warfare ~ and a shield bearing the
emblem of the future for the next generation of civilization
as it transitions into our future. She is symbolically adorned
head to toe. Grandmother Maria of Taos, New Mexico, USA,
original graphite, then colorized digitally in Australia by Beth
of Melbourne.

Page 18   **Purple**
by Beth of Australia

Page 19   **Abundance**
In our history of storytelling there is a mystical place that a
river flows thru the middle and at each bend gives food or
blankets. The representations tells that if we live a good life in
service to others and to our families that the reward exists to
show the reward that will come when a life of good has been
your walk upon Mother Earth. Grandmother Maria of Taos,
New Mexico, USA, original graphite, then colorized digitally
in Australia by Beth of Melbourne.

Page 21   **Weather Rock**
If the rock is white it is snowing if the rock is wet it's raining
if the rock is moving its windy.... The Red Tailed Hawk sitting
about represents the medicine of action. Graphite rendering
originally by Grandmother Maria of Taos, New Mexico, USA,
then digitally enhanced by Beth of Australia.

Page 23   **Tee Pee**
The home of the plains and some Southwest Indian tribes.
Its circular structure reflects the whole spiritual concept

of home and life "The Circle." Usually an individual family dwelling that comes with varying number of poles depending on the location of the tepee. Graphite rendering originally by Grandmother Maria of Taos, New Mexico,USA, then digitally enhanced by Beth of Australia.

Page 24   Animal Medicine
Colored Graphite originally conceived by Grandmother Maria of Taos, New Mexico, USA. Then digitally rendered by Two Feather to evolve into one of the first art pieces done in the beginning of the artistic phase of one person's life.

Page 27   Medicine Wheel
This depiction is to honor the Grandmothers & Grandfathers of the four directions. The three Eagle Feathers represents the two leggeds made up of the three aspects of people ~ Mind, Body & Spirit digitally rendered by Beth of Australia. This art piece took the better part of a month to intricately complete.

Page 28   Peacekeeper
Graphite rendering originally by Grandmother Maria of Taos, New Mexico, USA, then digitally enhanced by Beth of Australia.

Page 29   Innocence
Graphite rendering originally by Grandmother Maria of Taos, New Mexico, USA, then digitally enhanced by Beth of Australia.

Page 31   Unpredictability / Cougar
Graphite rendering originally by Grandmother Maria of Taos, New Mexico, USA, then digitally enhanced by Beth of Australia.

Page 32   A Medicine Shield
Depiction telling of a family background. Could be displayed near the entrance of dwelling area of some different tribal

systems. The number 3 that represents mind body and spirit is prominent in this art piece. Colored graphite by Grandmother Maria of Taos, New Mexico, USA ~ Digitally Enhanced by Two Feather.

Page 33   Red Tail Hawk
Digitally rendered and framed by Beth of Australia.

Page 35   The Beaver
Original graphite by Grandmother Maria of Taos, New Mexico, USA, and digitally enhanced and colorized by Beth of Australia.

Page 36   Healing
The mother snake represents healing as she weans the new borne into existence. This ancient Turtle Island symbol of healing in the way of a Caduceus style staff with 2 snakes with 3 heads upon it may have been the predecessor of the modern day American Medical Association AMA symbol? The item dominant in the top left is to honor our brothers and sisters from the stars referred to as "Star People." Set in the native turf of Two Feather ~ South West United States. Original Graphite by Grandmother Maria of Taos, New Mexico, USA. Digitally enhanced and colorized by Beth of Australia.

Page 37   The Deer
Original Graphite by Grandmother Maria of Taos, New Mexico, USA. Digitally enhanced and colorized by Beth of Australia.

Page 41   Swallow
Original by unknown Elders of long ago. Collected in the Grand Canyon area of Arizona, USA. Photo credits to William Two Feather 2008.

Page 42   Peace Bird in Flight
Colored graphite by Grandmother Maria of Taos, New
Mexico, USA. Digitally enhanced by Two Feather.

Page 43   Truth
Part of ones truth is what we own and that is what our
appaloosa pony can carry and we can handle, by this
measurement is truth. Original by Grandmother Maria of
Taos, New Mexico, USA . Digitally enhanced and colorized by
Beth of Australia.

Page 44   Bear In Water
Richard Dhalstrom from Cape Coral, Florida, USA.

Page 45   Bear
Original Graphite by Grandmother Maria of Taos, New
Mexico, USA. Digitally enhanced and colorized by Beth of
Australia.

Page 47   Raven
Colored art original graphite by Grandmother Maria of
Taos, New Mexico, USA and colorized by Beth of Australia..
Digitally enhanced by Two Feather.

Page 49   Snake
Digitally created and color enhanced by Beth of Australia

Page 50   Skin Caduceus
Original Graphite by Grandmother Maria of Taos, New
Mexico, USA. Digitally enhanced by William Two Feather
and colorized by Beth of Australia.

Page 51   Elk at Sunset
The Elk stands in the quiet Yosemite forest listening. Color
Pencil drawing by Nicole of San Diego, California, USA.

Page 52   Initiation

One spirit eagle materializes from the spirit realm to take a flesh offering of the riders chest then fades back into spirit world with the prize of initiation, willingly given. Then he comes to repeat the same taking of a flesh offering then to return to spirit world with his trophy as well. The turtle and red wolf accompany the seeker on his journey for support and guidance . Colored art original graphite by Grandmother Maria of Taos, New Mexico, USA. Colorized by Beth of Australia, digitally enhanced by Two Feather.

Page 53   Snow Goose

Original Graphite by Grandmother Maria of Taos, New Mexico, USA. Digitally enhanced by William Two Feather and colorized by Beth of Australia .

Page 55   Sturgeon

Original Graphite by Grandmother Maria of Taos, New Mexico, USA. Digitally enhanced and colorized by Beth of Australia.

Page 56   Mouse

Original by Sharon of Austin,Texas, USA, then digitally enhanced and colorized by Beth of Australia.

Page 57   Wolves

Original Graphite by Grandmother Maria of Taos, New Mexico, USA. Digitally enhanced and colorized by Beth of Australia.

Page 58   Wolverine

Original art by Nicole of San Diego, California, USA. Nicole is also in the healing arts as a practitioner and teacher.

Page 59   Turtle

Original Graphite by Grandmother Maria of Taos, New Mexico, USA. Digitally enhanced and colorized by Beth of Australia.

Page 70   Horses
Horses symbolize freedom and were the first transportation for the Plains People. It is a call to remember our own need to run free. Color pencil drawing by Nicole of San Diego, California, USA.

Page 71   Whispers
Original Graphite by Grandmother Maria of Taos, New Mexico, USA. Digitally enhanced and colorized by Beth of Australia.

Page 74   Yellow
Original graphic rendering by Beth of Australia.

Page 75   Red
Original graphic rendering by Beth of Australia.

Page 76   Black
Original graphic rendering by Beth of Australia.

Page 77   White
Original graphic rendering by Beth of Australia.

Page 78   Blue
Original graphic rendering by Beth of Australia.

Page 79   Purple
Original graphic rendering by Beth of Australia.

Page 80   Green
Original graphic rendering by Beth of Australia.

Page 81   "O"
Original graphic rendering by Beth of Australia.

Page 82   One
With-in all of us is the light and the dark. Which one we chose to feed is the one that will sit tall. Original Graphite

by Grandmother Maria of Taos, New Mexico, USA. Digitally enhanced and colorized by Beth of Australia.

Page 86   Shaman of The North
Richard D from Cape Coral, Florida, USA.

Page 87   The Embrace
Original Colored Graphite by Grandmother Maria of Taos, New Mexico, USA.

Page 89   Walk About
There are only two foreign art pieces in this book this is one of them. Speaks of how we are all related and as such should honor those different than us as if the were us. Originally digitally designed and conceived by Beth of Australia.

Page 90   Petroglyph Face
Original by unknown. Elders of long ago collected in the Grand Canyon area of Arizona, USA. Photo credits to William Two Feather 2008.

Page 92   Man
From Vallicitos, New Mexico, USA. Colored Graphite by Grandmother Maria of Taos, New Mexico, USA. Hidden in the scenery are many small wonders and treasures.

Page 93   Ghan Dancer
Richard D from Cape Coral, Florida, USA.

Page 91   Ancestors
The first people as we see it in Turtle Island were the Rock People. They have been here the longest of all of us and because of this we bestow upon them titles such as First People or Grandfathers. We seek their council in times of need. Original color pencil drawing by Nicole Desert Sage of San Diego, California, USA.

Page 111   Butterfly
A rare colorized art piece from Grandmother Maria of Taos,
New Mexico, USA. Originally a skeleton of black & white
graphite by Grandmother Maria of Taos, New Mexico, USA,
then magically colorized digitally in Australia by Beth of
Melbourne Australia.

Page 115   Sweat Lodge
Done by Kimba of San Diego, California, USA.
This art piece was fashioned from an actual Sweat lodge.
William Two Feather ran at a retreat for a few summer seasons
near Sedona, Arizona, USA, back before 2000. Kimba digitally
created this poster, USA .

Page 116   Teacher
Originally a skeleton of black & white graphite by
Grandmother Maria of Taos, New Mexico, USA then
magically colorized digitally in Australia by Beth of
Melbourne, Australia.

Page 118   Prayer
Originally a skeleton of black & white graphite by
Grandmother Maria of Taos, New Mexico, USA then
magically colorized digitally in Australia by Beth of
Melbourne, Australia.

Page 121   The Hunt
Originally a skeleton of black & white graphite by
Grandmother Maria of Taos, New Mexico, USA then
magically colorized digitally in Australia by Beth of
Melbourne, Australia

Page 123   The Medicine Wheel
Original black and white graphite by Grandmother Maria
of Taos, New Mexico, USA then colorized in Australia by
Beth of Melbourne, Australia. The Medicine Wheel is our
school room, chalk board and library all wrapped up into one

little symbol. The outer circle is the Grandfather Medicine (masculine) and the inner wheel is the hub the foundation and procreation (grandmother) medicine.

Page 124   Tree of Life
Original black and white graphite by Grandmother Maria of Taos, New Mexico, USA then colorized in Australia by Beth of Melbourne Australia. You may notice the varieties of fruits and sweets available from that which gives all for the people.

Page 126   The Chinupa & Buffalo
This digital rendition was compiled and rendered by Beth of Melbourne, Australia. The concept of this art piece is the path to world peace. If we sit in circles and pray together then where will the fight come from?

Page 127   Boy at Tree
Original pencil sketch by Paula Manning of Albuquerque, New Mexico, USA, then colorized and enhanced in Australia by Beth of Melbourne. All art takes time however each flower had to be intricately created and digitalized. The two feathers at each corner simultaneously honor the four directions and the two aspects with-in of all of us.

Page 130   Hummingbirds
A rare colorized art piece from Grandmother Maria of Taos, New Mexico, USA. As the ladies and maiden dance with their precious shawls ~ the humming birds bestow their beautiful blessings on them all. Set in my homelands the - Southwest USA.

Page 132   Hands Held High
Taken in New Mexico, USA. 2005. The two Buffalo skulls are used in certain ceremonies on a regular basis to honor the sacred place they have in our indigenous society. Sitting upon a buffalo robe tanned in the traditional way by means of the author by hand.

Page 136   Butterfly Woman
A rare colorized art piece from Grandmother Maria of Taos, New Mexico, USA. Represents 'turns for motions.'

Page 135   Warrior With Hawk
Richard D from Cape Corale, Florida, USA.

Page 137   Law of One
2006 Australia photo by "DV Photography," Australia. On a misty morning, Down Under, way out of town, we were on a small private lake. DV Photography has many accolades, locale in Australia and in many countries as well.

Page 138   Eagle Dance Boy
Original graphite by Paula Manning of Albuquerque, New Mexico, USA. Framed by Beth of Australia

Page 139   Oy Ya Te
Original black and white graphite by Grandmother Maria of Taos, New Mexico, USA then colorized in Australia by Beth of Melbourne, Australia.

Page 141   Matron Spirit Woman
Originally a skeleton of black and white graphite by Grandmother Maria of Taos, New Mexico, USA then magically colorized digitally in Australia by Beth of Melbourne, Australia. She is part of the wise woman series of patron spirits. Each is bejeweled with special attributes for purposes of prayer and communications to a specific ideal.

One voice when added to many becomes a mighty roar.

In 1977, human rights activist, Leonard Peltier, was unjustly convicted and imprisoned for the murder of two FBI agents which occured on the Pine Ridge Indian Reservation in 1975.

The persecution and subsequent conviction of Peltier were based on fabricated evidence, coerced testimonies and suppressed critical evidence.

Though these trial irregularities and many other inconsistencies have been bought to light, still this man remains behind bars, denied his rightful freedom and liberty and is considered by many throughout the world to be a political prisoner.

This obvious victimization and extreme lack of justice leaves a shameful stain on the United States of America as a country that prides itself on being a world leader of human rights, democracy, justice and freedom.

I urge each of you to seek your own knowledge of this case by visiting the various websites dedicated to Leonard. Then, if you believe an injustice has been committed against this man, pick up your pens and paper, and together with your conscience, write to the President of the United states of America asking for the release of Leonard Peltier.

Mr President
The White House
1600 Pennsylvania Avenue NW
Washington DC.
20500

Presidential Pardon

~ William Two Feather ~
www.2feather.com